THE TRUTH ABOUT SMOKING

SECOND EDITION

Robert N. Golden, M.D.
University of Wisconsin–Madison
General Editor

Fred L. Peterson, Ph.D.
University of Texas–Austin
General Editor

William McCay
Principal Author

Heath Dingwell, Ph.D.
Contributing Author

William Kane, Ph.D.
University of New Mexico
Adviser to the First Edition

Mark J. Kittleson, Ph.D.
Southern Illinois University
Adviser to the First Edition

Richelle Rennegarbe, Ph.D.
McKendree College
Adviser to the First Edition

Facts On File
An imprint of Infobase Publishing

The Truth About Smoking, Second Edition

Copyright © 2009 by DWJ BOOKS LLC

Facts On File, Inc.
An imprint of Infobase Publishing
132 West 31st Street
New York NY 10001

Library of Congress Cataloging-in-Publication Data

The truth about smoking / Robert N. Golden, general editor ... [et al.]. – 2nd ed.
    p. cm.
  Includes bibliographical references and index.
  ISBN-13: 978-0-8160-7632-1 (hardcover : alk. paper)
  ISBN-10: 0-8160-7632-4 (hardcover : alk. paper) 1. Smoking–Health aspects. 2. Tobacco use–Health aspects. I. Golden, Robert N.
  RA1242.T6M39 2009
  613.85–dc22   2008051963

Facts On File books are available at special discounts when purchased in bulk quantities for businesses, associations, institutions, or sales promotions. Please call our Special Sales Department in New York at (212) 967-8800 or (800) 322-8755.

You can find Facts On File on the World Wide Web at http://www.factsonfile.com

Text design by David Strelecky

Printed and bound in United States of America

MP MSRF 10 9 8 7 6 5 4 3 2 1

This book is printed on acid-free paper and contains 30 percent postconsumer recycled content.

CONTENTS

LIST OF ILLUSTRATIONS AND TABLES

PREFACE

The Truth About series—updated and expanded to include 20 volumes—seeks to identify the most pressing health issues and social challenges confronting our nation's youth. Adolescence is the period between the onset of puberty and the attainment of adult roles and responsibilities. Adolescence is also a time of storm, stress, and risk taking for many young people. During adolescence, a person's health is influenced by biological, psychological, and social factors, all of which interact with one's environment—family, peers, school, and community. It is a time when teenagers experience profound changes.

With the latest available statistics and new insights that have emerged from ongoing research, the Truth About series seeks to help young people build a foundation of information as they face some of the challenges that will affect their health and well-being. These challenges include high-risk behaviors, such as alcohol, tobacco, and other drug use; sexual behaviors that can lead to adolescent pregnancy and sexually transmitted diseases (STDs), such as HIV/AIDS; mental health concerns, such as depression and suicide; learning disorders and disabilities, which are often associated with school failures and school drop-outs; serious family problems, including domestic violence and abuse; and lifestyle factors, which increase adolescents' risk for noncommunicable diseases, such as diabetes and cardiovascular disease, among others.

Broader underlying factors also influence adolescent health. These include socioeconomic circumstances, such as poverty, available health care, and the political and social situations in which young people live. Although these factors can negatively affect adolescent health and well-being, as well as school performance, many of these negative health outcomes are preventable with the proper knowledge and information.

With prevention in mind, the writers and editors of each topical volume in the Truth About series have tried to provide cutting-edge information that is supported by research and scientific evidence. Vital facts are presented that inform youth about the challenges experienced during adolescence, while special features seek to dispel common myths and misconceptions. Some of the main topics explored include abuse, alcohol, death and dying, divorce, drugs, eating disorders, family life, fear and depression, rape, sexual behavior and unplanned pregnancy, smoking, and violence. All volumes discuss risk-taking behaviors and their consequences, healthy choices, prevention, available treatments, and where to get help.

In this new edition of the series, we also have added eight new titles in areas of increasing significance to today's youth. ADHD, or attention-deficit/hyperactivity disorder, and learning disorders are diagnosed with increasing frequency, and many students have observed or know of classmates receiving treatment for these conditions, even if they have not themselves received this diagnosis. Gambling is gaining currency in our culture, as casinos open and expand in many parts of the country, and the Internet offers easy access for this addictive behavior. Another consequence of our increasingly "online" society, unfortunately, is the presence of online predators. Environmental hazards represent yet another danger, and it is important to provide unbiased information about this topic to our youth. Suicide, which for many years has been a "silent epidemic," is now gaining recognition as a major public health problem throughout the life span, including the teenage and young adult years. We now also offer an overview of illness and disease in a volume that includes the major conditions of particular interest and concern to youth. In addition to illness, however, it is essential to emphasize health and its promotion, and this is especially apparent in the volumes on physical fitness and stress management.

It is our intent that each book serve as an accessible, authoritative resource that young people can turn to for accurate and meaningful answers to their specific questions. The series can help them research particular problems and provide an up-to-date evidence base. It is also designed with parents, teachers, and counselors in mind, so that they have a reliable resource that they can share with youth who seek their guidance.

Finally, we have tried to provide unbiased facts rather than subjective opinions. Our goal is to help elevate the health of the public with an emphasis on its most precious component—our youth. As young people face the challenges of an increasingly complex world, we as educators want them to be armed with the most powerful weapon available—knowledge.

Robert N. Golden, M.D.
Fred L. Peterson, Ph.D.
General Editors

HOW TO
USE THIS BOOK

NOTE TO STUDENTS

Knowledge is power. By possessing knowledge you have the ability to make decisions, ask follow-up questions, or know where to go to obtain more information. In the world of health that is power! That is the purpose of this book—to provide you the power you need to obtain unbiased, accurate information and *The Truth About Smoking.*

Topics in each volume of The Truth About are arranged in alphabetical order, from A to Z. Each of these entries defines its topic and explains in detail the particular issue. At the end of most entries are cross references to related topics. A list of all topics by letter can be found in the table of contents or at the back of the book in the index.

How have these books been compiled? First, the publisher worked with me to identify some of the country's leading authorities on key issues in health education. These individuals were asked to identify some of the major concerns that young people have about such topics. The writers read the literature, spoke with health experts, and incorporated their own life and professional experiences to pull together the most up-to-date information on health issues, particularly those of interest to adolescents and of concern in *Healthy People 2010.*

Throughout the alphabetical entries, the reader will find sidebars that separate Fact from Fiction. There are Question-and-Answer boxes that attempt to address the most common questions that youth ask about sensitive topics. In addition, readers will find a special feature called "Teens Speak"—case studies of teens with personal stories related to the topic in hand.

This may be one of the most important books you will ever read. Please share it with your friends, families, teachers, and classmates. Remember, you possess the power to control your future. One way to affect your course is through the acquisition of knowledge. Good luck and keep healthy.

NOTE TO LIBRARIANS

This book, along with the rest of The Truth About series, serves as a wonderful resource for young researchers. It contains a variety of facts, case studies, and further readings that the reader can use to help answer questions, formulate new questions, or determine where to go to find more information. Even though the topics may be considered delicate by some, don't be afraid to ask patrons if they have questions. Feel free to direct them to the appropriate sources, but do not press them if you encounter reluctance. The best we can do as educators is to let young people know that we are there when they need us.

Mark J. Kittleson, Ph.D.
Adviser to the First Edition

ADDICTIVE BEHAVIOR AND SMOKING

In the United States, smoking is still a problem at the societal level. Like gambling or overeating, smoking is an addictive behavior. However, there is good news. There has been a decrease in the number of people who smoke since the first edition of this book.

NEW IN THE REVISED EDITION

In this new edition of *The Truth About Smoking*, the statistics have been updated to reflect the most recent information available. For example, in 2002, smokers nationwide bought approximately 20 billion packs of cigarettes. By 2007, that number had dropped to 18.55 billion packs. That is 1.45 billion fewer cigarettes. It may not seem like much until the amount is spelled out: 1,450,000,000 fewer cigarettes.

The number of deaths from smoking-related illnesses has also dropped. In 2002, the Centers for Disease Control (CDC) reported that 440,000 people die from smoking-related illnesses. In 2007, that number dropped to 438,000 people. Once again, that may not seem like a big drop. To look at the figures from a different perspective, cities such as Rochester (N.Y.), Boise (Idaho), Spokane (Wash.), and Yonkers (N.Y.) each have populations close to 200,000.

Smoking continues to become more socially unacceptable. Smoking bans, often referred to as "clean air ordinances" are increasingly popular. Because most of these ordinances are passed at the local level, such as in towns and counties, it is difficult to determine how many exist. What has been determined is that these ordinances do not hurt businesses. It was feared that places such as restaurants and bars would lose money if customers could not smoke. However, research is consistently showing this is not the case.

To provide the latest information, six new articles have been added to this edition. These articles reflect concerns or issues important to teens. The first article or entry focuses on antismoking advocacy groups, such as the American Legacy Foundation, The Campaign for Tobacco-Free Kids, and Americans for Nonsmokers' Rights. You may be familiar with the truth® campaign. This campaign was begun in 2000 by the American Legacy Foundation. The campaign involves a series of edgy or provocative commercials that demonstrate how tobacco companies have lied about the harmful effects of smoking. Research now shows that these commercials have influenced teens' attitudes toward smoking.

Another entry focuses on the additive substances found in cigarettes. In order to make cigarettes easier to smoke and enjoy, companies add chemicals. For example, chemicals can alter the taste of cigarettes and make the smoke less painful when entering the lungs. However, cigarette company documents have indicated that additives were often used to increase the addictive nature of cigarettes. Chemicals such as ammonia and theobromine are added to increase the amount of nicotine absorbed into the body. This gives a smoker a stronger sensation, which increases the desire to continue smoking. Tobacco companies deny using chemicals to increase the addictiveness of cigarettes. As you will read, critics have presented evidence to the contrary.

Another article focuses on the cosmetic effects of smoking. Doctors have repeatedly shown that smoking damages the skin, teeth, hair, and a person's overall appearance. Smokers have skin that is more brittle, ages faster, and develops more wrinkles. Smokers are also more likely to lose their teeth and develop gum disease. Doctors also have shown that injuries take longer to heal in smokers. Smoking also causes teeth and fingernails to stain.

Two other entries are related to each other: the costs of smoking, and health insurance and smoking. Smokers spend more money on health care. Health insurance is extremely expensive. It can cost an employer more than $10,000 to provide health insurance to one employee and his or her family. Research has shown that smokers spend more money on health care. As a result, in an effort to keep insurance premiums down, some employers have employees pay a significant share of the health insurance premium, and some companies may refuse to hire, and may possibly fire, people who smoke.

The Centers for Disease Control estimate that smoking is responsible for more than $165 billion in health-care and disability costs every year. This is a large incentive for the government, insurance companies, and employers to help people kick the habit. At the same time, both state and federal governments make a tremendous amount of money from smokers. In 2005, approximately $82 billion was spent on cigarette purchases in the United States. For every pack of cigarettes sold, the state and federal governments collect taxes, which amounts to one-half of the price per pack.

The last article added to the new edition, "Tobacco Use and Socioeconomic Groups" focuses on the socioeconomic differences of smokers. Research shows that smokers are more likely to be less educated and earn less money than nonsmokers. Tobacco companies also spend more money on marketing toward lower-class groups. The assumption is that the wealthier and more educated members of society are better informed about the dangers of smoking. By comparison, those who earn less and are less educated are more likely to believe smoking is not addictive or dangerous. The unfortunate irony here is that the people who are most likely to smoke are the ones least likely to afford health insurance.

ADDICTIVE BEHAVIOR

Addiction is a condition in which a person habitually gives into a psychological or physical need for a substance such as alcohol, tobacco, or drugs. The substance becomes the focus of a person's life and begins to harm the individual or others physically, mentally, or socially. Addictive behavior includes psychological dependence on activities like overeating or gambling as well as physical addiction to chemicals like heroin or cocaine. Perhaps the thorniest discussion about addictive behavior is the ongoing argument about smoking cigarettes. Is tobacco use merely a bad habit that can be controlled and broken with a little willpower? Or is it a more serious problem with complex physical and psychological effects that keep smokers smoking?

Language purists complain that words like *addicted* and *addiction* are being stretched to cover so many situations that they're in danger of losing their original meanings. In a way, that has already happened.

Believe it or not, there was a time when addiction was a good thing. The word came into English more than 500 years ago as a legal term. Addiction occurred when people gave themselves over to a master to learn a trade as apprentices. Old books describe people as being addicted to learning or doing good works. By the 1800s, however, *addicted* began to refer more to harmful behaviors than to positive ones. Dictionaries used examples like "addicted to vice."

Then, approximately 100 years ago, doctors began writing about people giving themselves over to a new master—drugs. By 1951, *Webster's New Twentieth Century Dictionary* defined an addict as "one who is addicted, or strongly disposed to taking drugs." The 1960 *Webster's New Collegiate Dictionary* showed the beginnings of a new shift in meaning. An addict was defined as "one who is addicted to a habit, especially to the taking of some drug." In 1991, the Random House *Webster's College Dictionary* defined an addict as "one who is addicted to a substance, activity, or habit."

Do you see the change? People used to think that addiction required a physical substance. By the late 1900s, many recognized a psychological component to addiction as well. When someone can't stop buying shoes, it is not because something in the leather makes them addicted. Rather, some deep need is being met by the act of shopping, and satisfying that need has threatened people's jobs and destroyed their marriages.

An addict can be ruthless in acquiring whatever satisfies his or her **craving** or urge. Addicts will lie, cheat, or steal. They will manipulate people to get what they want. They'll be miserable and blame everyone but themselves if they can't feed their addiction. Far too much time goes into plotting how to get the all-important item, how to get it *now,* and even better, get more of it.

You might think the previous paragraph is somewhat dramatic when applied to a product that any adult can walk into a convenience store and buy. On the other hand, perhaps you have seen a 15-year-old one or two days after being cut off from his or her **nicotine** supply. Or you may consider this quotation from a 1969 presentation made to the board of directors at Philip Morris, one of the large tobacco companies: "Long after adolescent preoccupation with self-image has subsided, the cigarette will even preempt food in times of scarcity on the smoker's priority list."

THE CAUSE OF ADDICTION

Why would the top executives of a tobacco company expect hungry smokers to choose cigarettes over food? The answer is nicotine addiction. The nicotine in cigarettes is a powerful drug. Whether they realize it or not, smokers use nicotine to keep their stress levels down.

When they can't get nicotine, smokers become irritable and upset—a definite physical reaction. Cigarettes also have psychological value for smokers. Smoking offers a way of breaking the ice at parties or other social situations by offering someone a cigarette or asking for a light.

Unfortunately, cigarettes also have many negatives. Some of the really serious consequences of smoking take years to make themselves known.

You've probably heard the lectures and seen the pictures in health class. The worst part about smoking is that you're addicting yourself, giving yourself over to a master. You may be hooked before you even realize it. Only when you are scrambling to the store in the middle of the night because your pack ran out or lighting up when you are sick with the flu do you face the harsh realization that you no longer have a choice. You need that cigarette. And you need it *now*.

THE TOBACCO INDUSTRY

Imagine inventing a product that was inexpensive to make but for which people would pay almost anything to own and then keep coming back for more. Increase that business to an almost unimaginable scale, and you begin to approach the business position of **Big Tobacco**, the half-dozen major corporations that control the production and sale of tobacco products around the world. Papers recently acquired from these companies show that the production cost varies greatly depending on whom you ask: R.J. Reynolds states $1.38 a pack, while the New York State Quitline reports $0.05. Compare that to the retail cost at a local store. Admittedly, tobacco companies face additional expenses. The cigarettes have to be stored and shipped. Distribution costs add to the price, as do federal, state, and local taxes. Even with these added costs, tobacco companies make a handsome profit.

Going back to our hypothetical "must-have" product, imagine making 24 cents a day from one-quarter of the people in your neighborhood, country, or state.

Although it appears that anyone would be happy to own the company producing our imaginary product, this remarkable moneymaking product causes a serious illness or death to a substantial percentage of its users. Again, according to the Centers for Disease Control and Prevention, 438,000 Americans die each year from smoking-related illnesses.

Cigarettes became a big business in the 1880s. Tobacco companies enjoyed ever-growing sales—and profits—through the 1940s. In the 1950s, however, news stories began to appear reporting that researchers were finding health problems connected with smoking, including cancer.

This research came as a shock to the executives who ran the tobacco corporations. Up to that point, they thought their product offered an inexpensive pleasure to millions of people. Drawbacks seemed minor. Some smokers complained of coughs and sore throats. Others lost their breath more easily than nonsmokers. While not exactly healthy, cigarettes didn't seem harmful. Tobacco companies used such advertising lines as, "Not a cough in a carload" and promoted their products as "smooth" or "mild."

If cigarettes were found to have serious, even fatal, side effects, tobacco companies wouldn't just lose sales. They could be sued for selling a dangerous product and face financial ruin.

The companies instituted their own research to eliminate the dangerous ingredients in tobacco smoke and make their products safer, an effort that continues today. At the same time, Big Tobacco tried to sweep the bad news under the rug until they could rectify matters.

Tobacco companies spent considerable time, effort, and money challenging the unfavorable research findings by raising questions about the research. Competing companies joined forces to create and fund the TIRC (Tobacco Industry Research Committee, also known as the Tobacco Institute and the Council for Tobacco Research), an industry group whose only job was to convince the public that scientists were not sure if smoking was dangerous. Whenever new research connected smoking to health risks, this group would fire off press releases to debate the value of these discoveries.

The strategy created a controversy fought in the media, with claims and counterclaims running in newspapers and magazines and also on radio and television. The TIRC combed scientific journals for research that bolstered the tobacco companies' position and publicized that research as loudly as possible. Press releases and fact sheets went out to influential editors and publishers. The group even hired writers to create articles that "proved" cigarettes were safe. The media war continued even as research sponsored by the tobacco companies verified the findings of independent researchers.

Over three decades, the TIRC became so well-known—or infamous—that it was forced out of existence as part of a legal settlement in 1998. But the group succeeded in creating a "tobacco controversy," confusing a lot of people who kept buying cigarettes.

To date, the "safer" tobacco products that have hit the market turned out to be more about public relations than public health. The cover-up continues today.

In 2004 many Americans marked the 40th anniversary of what people call the "first surgeon general's report." The **surgeon general** is the nation's highest government health official. He or she heads the U.S. Public Health Service. In 1962, Surgeon General Luther Terry gathered a committee of scientists and health experts to examine the evidence linking smoking with various diseases. Terry asked the cigarette companies for their research so the committee could make an informed decision. The cigarette manufacturers gave limited information, significantly damaging data.

One may speculate as to what the world would be like if the tobacco companies' information had been released in the 1960s instead of leaked to the press in the 1990s. Would cigarette sales have dropped more rapidly? Since 1965, tobacco's most successful year, sales have consistently shown a decline. Would there have been lawsuits? The tobacco companies have kept their lawyers busy for years, contesting cases brought by people who became ill or died because of cigarettes. Internal records discovered or leaked because of these cases have only made the corporations look worse.

THE TOBACCO CONTROVERSY

For 40 years, controversy has swirled around a major American business, getting sharper and nastier, it seems, with every decade. Some people complain about the shrill tone of the antismoking forces. Part of that shrillness comes from trying to be heard. A 2006 report by the California Department of Health Services indicated that the tobacco industry spends 20 times more money on advertising and marketing than the state of California spends on tobacco-education programs. The state spent $3.44 per person on tobacco education, while the tobacco industry spent $69.75 per person on advertising and marketing efforts.

If the tobacco companies keep a calm tone in their public relations, they also have a long history of funding supposedly "independent" groups to attack and vilify opponents. An incident in the late 1990s illustrates the extent of the problem. At the time, some tobacco companies admitted on their corporate web sites that their products caused health problems. The immediate reaction was suspicion. "What are they up to? Why did their lawyers tell them to do that?" people asked. After 40 years of evasion, this general distrust of Big Tobacco is like a sore that never heals—a cancer, if you like, on American public life.

THE IMPACT ON SOCIETY

Consider a snapshot of the United States as it was about a century ago. According to statistics from the American Lung Association, cigarette manufacturers sold 2.5 billion cigarettes in 1900. (Today, production is closer to 371 billion.) Most Americans in 1900 preferred to chew their tobacco rather than smoke it. An Internet web site on tobacco history (www.sweducationcenter.org) reports that 58 percent of the tobacco consumed in the United States in 1900 was chewed. Only 1 percent was smoked as cigarettes.

In 1900, lung cancer was an extremely rare disease, and few people died of heart attacks. This was an era in which many people died young from diseases that are controlled today, like tuberculosis. The average lifespan was much shorter.

Doctors began seeing a rise in lung cancer after American participation in World War I (1917–1919). When American troops marched off to war, their rations included free cigarettes. For many young men, this was their introduction to smoking. Many remained committed smokers for the rest of their lives.

Even in the 1930s, lung cancer was a comparatively rare condition. However, the death toll from this disease would rise sharply over the next 60 years, even as new treatments reduced mortality rates for other forms of cancer.

During those years, young men once again went off to war (World War II, 1941–1945) with cigarettes in their rations. Again, many servicemen came home as confirmed smokers. The number of smokers continued to rise through the mid-1960s. In 1965, more than half of the adult males in the United States smoked. Fifteen to twenty years later, the cancer rate soared.

Speaking at the release of the 40th surgeon general's report in 2004, Surgeon General Richard H. Carmona noted that more than 12 million people have died from smoking-related illness since the first surgeon general's report in 1964. These deaths include 4.1 million deaths from cancer, 5.5 million deaths from cardiovascular diseases (heart attacks and **strokes**), 2.1 million deaths from respiratory diseases, and 94,000 infant deaths. Carmona warned that nearly 25 million Americans alive today will die prematurely unless they quit smoking cigarettes.

Death rates from smoking-related diseases rose even as the number of Americans who smoked decreased. Statistics from the World Health Organization, the international public health agency of the United Nations, show that smoking is on the decline in the United States, Canada, Japan, and most of the developed nations in northern and western Europe. For most of the world, however, the number of smokers is still rising. How will poor countries that don't have enough hospitals for current medical problems deal with a flood of patients with smoking-related illnesses in the future?

In terms of treatment costs and lost productivity from sick or deceased patients, the United States has paid a terrible price for the popularity of smoking. The American economy has been strong enough to survive the impact, but many of the places where smoking is on the rise are poor countries like Bangladesh or countries still developing their economies like Malaysia. How will these nations cope with the costs of a huge public-health crisis? Who can predict the economic and political results?

FACING THE FUTURE

While reviewing the state of smoking in 2004, Surgeon General Carmona also reflected on the government's hopes for the future. He and other public health leaders have set ambitious goals for the coming decade. They hope to reduce the percentage of smokers to 12 percent from the present number of 20.8 percent. Accomplishing that objective would save more than seven million Americans from premature death.

The task, Carmona admitted, is difficult. Unless more people can be persuaded to quit smoking, the rate of deaths related to the habit will not decline for many years to come. The percentage of smokers in the population has held fairly steady in recent years. Some suggest that those who have not quit represent hard-core smokers, those who are most determined to stay with the habit—or those who are most addicted.

As new research reveals the dangers of secondhand smoke—smoke discharged into the air by cigarettes and smokers—attitudes are hardening among nonsmokers. Instead of a nuisance, smoke in the air is increasingly viewed as a health hazard. Smokers may choose to risk their health—that is their right. If the ingredients in cigarette smoke that cause illness in smokers also affect those around them, nonsmokers should have the right to insist on a smoke-free environment.

Smoking has been such a part of the American scene for so long that many simply take the act of smoking for granted. Surveys show that over the years, however, nonsmokers are becoming less and less tolerant of smoking, and there are three nonsmoking American adults for every smoker.

Facing the future is also a personal challenge. The catchphrase "Young people are our future" may be a cliché, but it is also the truth. Most smokers start when they are young, and many smokers are young people. The decision to smoke can affect a person's future. In some cases, it can make that future drastically shorter. As a smoker, a friend of a smoker, or someone who is tempted to explore smoking, you must be aware that a choice made now can have consequences for decades to come.

With the information in this book, you should find enough facts to make an informed decision about smoking. And if you're presently smoking, you may get enough facts to do more than just consider stopping.

Before you start taking on those facts, however, why not discover what you already know about the subject of smoking?

RISKY BUSINESS SELF-TEST

As you answer true or false to the following statements, keep a record of your answers on a sheet of paper so that you can assess your knowledge of the facts.

Twenty questions about smoking and smokers

Look over these statements about tobacco. Identify whether each is true or false.

1. Smoking is just a bad habit.
2. Smoking helps you concentrate.
3. Most children of smokers hate smoking.
4. Ads don't really convince people to smoke.
5. Smoking cigarettes leads to more serious drugs.
6. Lots of people smoke—just take a look at the movies.
7. Smoking can take almost 15 years off a woman's life.

8. Smoking is a favorite method of relaxation for the rich and famous.

9. The percentage of smokers does not vary from one ethnic group to another.

10. Smoking doubles the risk for a heart attack.

11. Two-thirds of students in high school have tried smoking.

12. It's easier for an alcoholic to stop drinking than it is for a smoker to stop smoking.

13. Cigarettes are just tobacco and paper.

14. Kids under age 12 just play at smoking.

15. Most smokers enjoy smoking. Otherwise, why would they do it?

16. Smokers are 10 times more likely to get lung cancer than nonsmokers.

17. When people quit smoking, they gain weight.

18. Using smokeless tobacco is safer than smoking.

19. The information about the effects of secondhand smoke is just a scare tactic.

20. Smoking is just a phase kids go through.

The answers

1. False. The nicotine in tobacco is addictive. People suffer withdrawal symptoms when they attempt to quit smoking.

2. True. Better concentration, even in noisy environments, seems to be one of the few positive effects of nicotine.

3. False. Children of smokers are twice as likely to become smokers as the children of nonsmokers.

4. False. Tobacco companies claim that advertising only convinces smokers which brand to choose. Historically, however, significant rises in tobacco use have followed major, innovative ad campaigns.

5. True. For some, smoking is the first step in a series of risky choices. Researchers on drug abuse at Columbia University discovered that nine out of 10 cocaine users started out as smokers.

6. False. Less than 25 percent of adult Americans smoke. Most people, including most young people, do not smoke.

7. True. According to life expectancy studies by the Centers for Disease Control and Prevention, women who smoke can expect on average to live 14.5 years less than female nonsmokers.

8. False. Despite glamorous images in the media, the highest percentage of smokers in the United States can be found among high school dropouts and the unemployed.

9. False. Surveys show that different ethnic groups have different smoking habits. Native Americans and Alaska Natives have the highest percentages of smokers in the United States. Statistically, Asian Americans smoke less than the national average. Caucasian Americans tend to smoke more than African Americans or Latinos.

10. True. This is just one of an array of alarming statistics about the impact of tobacco smoke on the cardiovascular system. Smoking has many bad effects on the heart and blood vessels, including stroke and hardening of the arteries.

11. False. The most recent statistic for students who tried smoking was 46.2 percent. Fewer high school students are actual smokers, however.

12. True. Recent research shows that sensitivity to alcohol and nicotine may be genetic—it may run in people's families. However, while statistics show that many alcoholics manage to stop drinking, they continue to smoke.

13. False. Companies add some 600 chemicals to cigarettes to flavor them and even to make them burn evenly. Scientists have identified more than 4,000 chemicals

in cigarette smoke. About 43 of those chemicals are known to cause cancer.

14. False. A full 8 percent of middle school students have completely smoked a cigarette before the age of 11. People who start smoking at a young age typically spend more years smoking and have greater difficulty in quitting.

15. False. Government surveys find that nearly 70 percent of smokers were interested in quitting. Nearly one-half (46 percent) attempt to quit each year, but the success rate is under 10 percent. According to the American Heart Association, the key to success is not giving up. People who keep trying to quit have a 50–50 chance of success.

16. True. The American Lung Association warns that one in three smokers will die early. Smokers face much higher rates for disorders of the lungs, heart, and the blood vessels. They also suffer a higher rate for cancers in other parts of the body, such as the stomach, bladder, kidneys, and even certain types of leukemia.

17. True. Nicotine does depress the appetite, but it will not keep weight off. Inactive smokers can expect to gain about five pounds on average if they quit smoking. Some studies indicate that women tend to gain more weight than men after they stop smoking. By no means should weight gain be an excuse for not trying to quit. After beating nicotine, working off a few extra pounds shouldn't be difficult at all. A 15-minute walk each day should be enough to burn the necessary calories.

18. False. Although smokeless tobacco users are at lower risk for lung cancer, they have a greater risk of developing oral (mouth) cancer. Approximately 30,000 people a year die from oral cancer. Three-quarters of those deaths can be linked to the use of smokeless tobacco. People who develop oral cancer undergo often disfiguring surgery to remove **tumors**, losing parts of their face, jaw, and tongue.

19. False. Some 3,000 nonsmoking Americans die of lung cancer each year from breathing other people's cigarette smoke. Tests of blood, urine, and hair of nonsmokers who spend time in environments with cigarette smoke reveal breakdown products of nicotine in the systems of nonsmokers. Hair tests on newborn babies show that the developing baby can be exposed to nicotine if the mother or other people around her smoke cigarettes during the pregnancy.

20. False. The American Legacy Foundation, an antismoking group, conducted a long-term study on teenagers and smoking. Only 5 percent of the teens questioned thought they would be smoking in five years. Yet when researchers checked in with them eight years later, 75 percent of the study subjects were still smoking. Other research finds 90 percent of lifetime smokers begin before their 18th birthdays. These long-time smokers also have a much more difficult time trying to quit.

KNOWING THE SCORE

Were you able to tell fact from fiction? How many answers did you already know? How many surprised you?

As you look through the various entries in the rest of this book, expect to find more surprises. Even some well-informed adults who looked over the manuscript found facts that challenged things they'd always believed—things that "everybody knows."

That's the annoying thing about facts. You have to keep picking them up, expanding your knowledge. When it comes to questions of your health, however, you don't have a choice. What you don't know *can* hurt—and even kill you.

A TO Z ENTRIES

■ ADDICTION, PRODUCTS TO OVERCOME

A condition in which a person habitually gives into a psychological or physical need for a substance such as tobacco is called addiction. After years of studying why smokers continue to smoke, researchers have identified nicotine, a substance in tobacco and tobacco smoke, as an addictive substance. In recent years, a number of products have been introduced to help smokers overcome their addiction to nicotine. A bad habit can be broken with willpower alone, but a person fighting an addiction is likely to need additional assistance.

NICOTINE REPLACEMENT

When asked about the biggest obstacle to quitting, 70 to 90 percent of smokers mention withdrawal symptoms. Cutting off their usual flow of nicotine makes smokers irritable and nervous. Often they have difficulty concentrating. **Nicotine replacement therapy** consists of products such as the nicotine patch, gum, nasal spray, inhalers, and lozenges. Each supplies those who are trying to quit smoking with enough nicotine to relieve their worst symptoms. These products help take the edge off cravings without exposing anyone to cancer-causing tars and poisonous gases found in tobacco smoke. They provide an alternative to going "cold turkey"—trying to stop smoking with no help at all.

Nicotine replacement starts when smoking stops. A person should not smoke while using nicotine patches, gums, or nasal sprays. The whole idea is to establish a level of nicotine that lets a user feel reasonably comfortable and then to reduce the dose in several stages. Smoking while using nicotine replacements might raise nicotine levels in the body to a dangerous point.

Nicotine replacement or stop-smoking products can be just as expensive as cigarettes in the short term, although the Internet allows people to find some more cost-effective options. How successful are these products? It depends on the product. In a 2006 article in *American Family Physician,* researchers compared the effectiveness of several products. Specifically, the authors wanted to see how many people still refrained from smoking six months after starting the therapy.

Among those who relied on self-help materials, between 7 and 27 percent of smokers had remained smoke-free six months later.

Between 21 and 30 percent of people using Bupropion remained smoke-free after six months. Thirty percent of individuals using a nicotine spray also remained smoke-free after six months. Nicotine gum and lozenges appeared to be equally effective, with 24 percent of users remaining smoke-free at the six month mark.

Combination therapies proved to be the most effective. Between 8 and 21 percent of smokers who used a nicotine patch alone were still smoke-free after six months. However, when adding a nicotine spray, 37 percent of smokers remained smoke-free after three months. (Quit rates at the six month mark were not available for this treatment combination.) Combining the patch and Bupropion also was effective—35 percent of smokers remained smoke-free after six months when using these therapies.

Fact Or Fiction?

If you're someplace where they don't allow you to smoke, bring along some nicotine gum.

The Facts: Nicotine replacement products are intended to help smokers quit, not to help them keep smoking.

At this point, no one is sure what the long-term effects of nicotine products are. Doctors recommend that people use nicotine replacement for three or six months. Even though products are sold over-the-counter, they are still medicine.

The patch

The nicotine transdermal system, better known as the patch, is an adhesive bandage containing nicotine. This nonprescription nicotine replacement transmits a measured dose of the drug through the wearer's skin. The patch looks like a large bandage, about three inches across. The user peels the backing off and smoothes the patch on a clean section of nonhairy skin between the neck and the waist or on an arm. The patch cannot be used on broken, cut, or irritated skin. Each time it is changed, the patch should be placed in a new location. Some patches stay on for 16 hours and come off at night. Others are replaced every 24 hours. Users are warned to keep new and used patches away from children and pets. The nicotine can be poisonous to small children and animals.

Possible side effects from nicotine patches include headache, dizziness, blurred vision, and vivid dreams. Many people experience itching, burning, and redness on the skin beneath the patch, which is why users must keep moving their patches around. The full treatment lasts two months to 10 weeks, with users stepping down the dosage in several stages.

The patch can be purchased without a prescription, but it's best to talk to a doctor before starting, especially if the prospective user is under 18 years of age. The patch can interfere with certain medicines and adversely affect some medical conditions. A doctor should know if the person intending to use the patch has a history of heart problems, diabetes, liver or kidney disease, or allergies to tape, bandages, or medicines.

Users should be aware of the possibility of overdosing, especially if they continue to smoke cigarettes while wearing the patch. Symptoms of nicotine overdose include cold sweat, dizziness, nausea, drooling, confusion, and even fainting. The doctor should be called immediately in such a situation.

Because the brain isn't used to dealing with nicotine during sleeping hours, users of the 24-hour patch may experience strange dreams or sleeplessness. Users of the 16-hour patch may have to deal with morning cravings for a cigarette. Because the patch delivers a steady dose of nicotine, it can't help users to deal with sudden cravings for a cigarette.

Q & A

Question: Who can I talk to if I think I might have a smoking problem?

Answer: Talk to your doctor or your dentist. You might also check state or local health agencies for programs that help smokers quit. You can find them in the blue pages of the phone book. Most libraries have information as well. You may also want to speak with your parents, a school counselor, or a religious leader in your community. If you think you need help, it's a good idea to start looking for it.

Nicotine gum

Chewing a nicotine gum offers another nonprescription method for delivering nicotine into the body. The nicotine enters the bloodstream through the membranes in the mouth.

Those who choose to use a nicotine gum need special instructions for chewing the product to ensure that they release the nicotine correctly. The idea is to chew only until a "peppery" taste or a tingle in the mouth indicate that the nicotine has been released. The user then "parks" the gum at the side of the mouth, between the gum and the cheek, where it acts like an internal patch, transferring nicotine through the inner cheek. As the tingle fades, the user chews again, exposing a new piece of the gum and releasing additional nicotine.

Too much chewing or too vigorous a chewing action can free nicotine too quickly, leading to an overdose or stomach problems if the nicotine is swallowed. One piece of gum should last for about 30 minutes. When the user no longer feels a tingle, it's time to discard the gum. Again, care should be taken to keep used gum away from children and pets.

People using the gum follow a regular schedule, chewing a piece or two of gum every one to two hours. In the event of a sudden craving they can chew an additional piece to blunt the compulsion. On average, users chew 10–15 pieces per day, with a maximum of 30 if necessary. After stabilizing for a month, users begin to reduce the number of pieces chewed each day until they only chew when they experience withdrawal symptoms. The treatment is supposed to last about three months, but some users have relied on the gum for six months or even a year.

Although nicotine gum is available without a prescription, smokers who wish to use the gum to quit would be wise to consult their doctors before starting a program, particularly if the prospective users are under the age of 18.

The advantage of nicotine gum is that it can be used to respond quickly to cravings. The gum works more slowly than a cigarette, however, and the nicotine dose is lower. Users shouldn't eat or drink for 15 minutes before using the gum or while they are chewing it. Acidic food and beverages such as coffee, fruit juices, and soda can affect how well the gum works by changing the chemical balance in the mouth, which in turn affects how well the nicotine is absorbed.

Other drawbacks to nicotine gum include a bad taste, aching jaws from constant chewing, a sore throat, and even sores in the throat and mouth. Swallowing nicotine in saliva can cause hiccups and upset the stomach. If a user should actually swallow the gum, he or she may risk a nicotine overdose. Anyone swallowing the gum should see a doctor or visit the local poison control center.

Some researchers are experimenting with a mixed nicotine replacement therapy, using the patch to provide a steady dose of nicotine with a limited supply of nicotine gum for emergency use against strong cravings.

Those who use nicotine gum should also read and carefully follow the instructions that come with the product. Besides explaining how to use the gum, the instructions also offer useful quitting tips.

Nasal spray

Another nicotine delivery system used by people who want to stop smoking is a nasal spray. Users spray a controlled dose up each nostril. The nicotine is then absorbed into the bloodstream through the skin of the nasal membranes. Nicotine nasal sprays come in pump bottles, each containing about 100 doses of nicotine in a water-based solution. A dose in this case means a single spray up each nostril. Each dose is equivalent to the amount of nicotine in

DID YOU KNOW?

Percentage of Smokers Using Various Quitting Methods and Their Success Rates, 2000

	Preferred Method %	Success Rates %
Cold turkey/self-help	90.4	<10.0
Counseling/behavioral	1.3	15.0
Nicotine replacement therapy		
Nicotine patch	4.2	17.7
Nicotine gum	1.6	23.7
Nasal spray	0	30.5
Nicotine inhaler	<1.0	22.8
Non-nicotine therapy		
Bupropion	1.2	30.5

Source: National Health Interview Survey, 2000.

one cigarette. The nicotine spray is the fastest delivery system for nicotine replacement.

Those trying to quit smoking use the spray once or twice each waking hour, with additional sprays if they have to fight cravings—up to a maximum of 40 doses a day. Users complain that the spray can sting at first. Other negative effects include watery eyes, sneezing, coughing, nosebleeds, a sudden rapid heartbeat, and diarrhea. The spray is not recommended for people with nasal or sinus problems, asthma, or allergies.

The spray's greatest advantage is the speed it offers to users in responding to cravings. Users also have more control over doses than with other nicotine replacement methods. On the other hand, in some situations using a spray may not be convenient. Nicotine spray can also become addictive. It's the hardest replacement therapy to stop. For these reasons, people need a doctor's prescription to use it. The Food and Drug Administration (FDA), the federal agency in charge of drug safety, recommends that the spray be used only for three months—six months at the most.

ADDITIONAL PRODUCTS

Another prescription nicotine replacement system is the nicotine inhaler, a tube with a nicotine cartridge inside. A user puffs on the tube, bringing nicotine into the mouth, where it is absorbed through the skin. Those trying to quit may prefer the inhaler because puffing on it closely resembles actually smoking. However, inhalers are the most expensive form of replacement therapy.

Some people prefer a nicotine replacement therapy that offers the drug in lozenge form. A user absorbs the nicotine through the skin of the mouth while sucking on a hard candy. The product is used in a 12-week program. For the first six weeks, users take a lozenge every one to two hours. Over the course of the next three weeks, they cut the dosage down to one lozenge every two to four hours. In the final three weeks of the program, users take a lozenge every four to eight hours.

As with nicotine gum, lozenges must be taken in a special way. In the 20 to 30 minutes it takes for the lozenge to dissolve, a user must move it from side to side in the mouth. Most experience a tingle as the nicotine is absorbed. It is important not to swallow while letting the lozenge dissolve. Swallowing nicotine-laced saliva can cause hiccups and upset the stomach. Users are also warned not to chew on the lozenges; doing so may release a larger than desirable dose of nicotine.

Although the lozenges are available without a prescription, users must be over the age of 18. As with the patch and nicotine gum, those interested in the product are advised to consult a doctor before starting the therapy.

NON-NICOTINE REPLACEMENT THERAPY

Bupropion is a prescription medicine originally developed to help people suffering from depression. The drug is marketed under the brand name Welbutrin as an antidepression medicine and under the name **Zyban** to help smokers quit.

A major test conducted by the University of Wisconsin School of Medicine compared the effectiveness of nicotine replacement with the new drug. The results were published in the March 4, 1999, issue of the *New England Journal of Medicine.* In this test of 893 smokers, one group used Zyban alone, another used it along with the nicotine patch, and a third group used only the patch. A fourth group was given a **placebo,** a pill containing no medication administered for its psychological effect. A year later, 30.3 percent of the participants who used Zyban alone remained smoke-free. Those receiving the Zyban-patch combination had a success rate of 35.5 percent. Participants using the patch only or the placebo had success rates of 16.4 percent and 15.6 percent respectively.

Zyban is a prescription drug. Before prescribing it, doctors often require a check-up and a full medical history, including all other drug use by the patient. Zyban may interact with other medications for depression, for instance. Another important consideration is whether the patient or the patient's family has a history of seizures. In a seizure, the brain's electrical activity becomes disturbed, creating muscular spasms and causing a person to lose control of body movements. A very small percentage of Zyban users may suffer seizures which could be life-threatening. Thus, people who are subject to seizures should not use the drug.

In 2006, the FDA approved another medication to help people quit smoking. Varenicline, marketed under the name Chantix, was developed solely to help smokers quit. The drug targets the same receptors in the brain as nicotine. As a result, nicotine withdrawal symptoms are reduced. At the same time, the drug reduces the pleasurable effects of smoking. Because Chantix is so new, it is too early to determine exactly its effectiveness. A study by Pfizer, the manufacturer of Chantix, found that 44 percent of the people taking Chantix quit smoking. In 2006, two studies appeared in the *Journal of the American Medical Association.* Both studies found that Chantix was more effective than Zyban in helping smokers quit.

In 2007, the FDA started to issue warnings about the use of Chantix because of reports that people were having negative reactions to the drug. These reactions included agitation, anxiety, depression, suicidal thoughts, and suicide attempts. Doctors have been urged to closely monitor their patients who are on Chantix. More research is needed to fully determine the safety of this new smoking cessation drug.

A MAJOR CHANGE

Even as recently as 25 years ago, people were still arguing over the addictive properties of nicotine. Final recognition that nicotine is addictive—and that smoking is an addiction—has changed the outlook for people trying to quit. Treatments have been developed that are both medically approved and socially acceptable.

A smoker trying to quit can now blunt cravings with a variety of products that will deliver a dose of nicotine without cancer-causing chemicals. Smokers can also use a non-nicotine treatment—a prescription pill which counteracts nicotine cravings. With these therapies, smokers have a much better chance to break the hold of a dependency that is far more than a habit.

See also: Addiction to Nicotine; Body and Smoking, The

FURTHER READING

Brizer, David. *Quitting Smoking for Dummies.* New York: Wiley, 2003.

Miller, Barbara. *How to Quit Smoking Even if You Don't Want To.* Victoria, B.C., Canada: Trafford Publishing, 2006.

Whetherall, Charles. *Quit: Read This Book and Stop Smoking.* Philadelphia, Pa.: Running Press Miniature Editions, 2007.

■ ADDICTION TO NICOTINE

Nicotine is an addicting agent found in tobacco plants. A natural poison, nicotine protects tobacco plants from bugs. A large enough dose of nicotine—40 to 60 milligrams, the equivalent of a few drops—can kill a grown person. If a few drops of the pure poison touch mucous tissues (such as the damp skin inside the mouth or nose), the person can die. People have actually been murdered through nicotine poisoning.

For years, debate raged over whether nicotine was an addictive substance. One might think the matter would have been settled when Surgeon General C. Everett Koop, the highest medical authority in the nation, issued a report in 1988 titled, "The Health Consequences of Smoking: Nicotine Addiction." Yet as recently as 1994, tobacco executives claimed that nicotine was not addictive.

Today, Philip Morris, a major tobacco corporation, states on its web site that the company "agrees with the overwhelming medical and scientific consensus that cigarette smoking is addictive. It can be very difficult to quit smoking." Nicotine is the major reason why people smoke and why they continue to smoke, year after year.

PHYSIOLOGICAL EFFECTS OF NICOTINE

Nicotine can enter the body in several ways. It "hitches a ride" into the lungs by attaching to tar, the tiny solid particles in tobacco smoke. People who smoke pipes and cigars do not draw smoke into their lungs. Instead, those who use smokeless tobacco acquire nicotine through the mucous membranes in the mouth.

Once inside the body, nicotine enters a complicated chemical communications system. The body has three basic varieties of message-bearing chemicals. **Cytokines** stir up or suppress the mechanisms of the immune system to deal with invading bacteria and viruses. **Hormones** transmit messages to start or stop activity in organs or tissues, controlling blood pressure, the production of red blood cells, the amount of sugar in the blood, and regulating the salt and water balance in the body, among many other activities. Finally, **neurotransmitters** carry messages through the spaces between nerve cells, or between nerve and muscle cells. All these chemicals allow the various organs to communicate with one another and help the body as a whole to function.

Neurotransmitters help messages travel along nerves. These messages may be reports of sensations, orders to muscles, information about various parts of the body, or orders to produce hormones. Whatever the message, information passes through a nerve cell as an electrical impulse. Neurotransmitters carry the message between

DID YOU KNOW?

Percent of People 18 or Older Who Smoked, Select Years, 1965–2005

	Total %	Sex	
		% Male	% Female
1965	50.1	28.9	21.1
1970	48.1	26.4	21.6
1974	48.9	25.8	23.1
1980	51.6	27.5	24.1
1985	50.4	25.7	24.7
1990	45.8	24.2	21.6
1995	47.2	24.7	22.6
2000	46.5	24.6	21.9
2005	45.1	24.8	20.3
Percent change 1965–2005	−10.0	−14.2	−3.8

As this table shows, smoking has declined since 1965.

Source: American Lung Association, 2007.

nerve cells. The transmitting ends of the cell store as many as 10,000 tiny chemical molecules. There are about 50 different varieties, depending on the message being sent. Thousands of these neurotransmitters spread out across the space between nerve cells. The surface of the next cell is covered with molecules called receptor sites. Each receptor site accepts only one variety of neurotransmitter, just as a lock receives a key. Depending on which receptor is "unlocked," a particular message is passed along.

Another system, the blood-brain barrier, is supposed to protect the brain from toxic chemicals in the body. The problem is that nicotine gets past this defense. Its molecular structure mimics one of the body's natural neurotransmitters. Once it's in the bloodstream, nicotine travels to the brain, binds to receptor sites there, and sets off a chain of reactions, the basic nicotine cycle.

The nicotine stimulates production of the hormone epinephrine, a form of adrenaline, which usually acts to put the body on alert in life-or-death situations. The hormone causes a surge of insulin, releasing sugar into the blood and creating a burst of energy. As the nicotine level in the body decreases, so does the sugar. The smoker feels depressed and tired—and lights another cigarette. That's the basic nicotine cycle, but much more goes on in the body.

Epinephrine revs up other body functions as preparation for great exertion. Both breathing and heartbeat become faster, putting stress on the lungs and heart. Blood vessels constrict, making blood pressure rise. Most importantly, nicotine activates the parts of the brain involved with pleasure. It releases the "feel-good" neurotransmitter, dopamine, the same reaction that occurs when addictive drugs like cocaine or heroin enter the body.

Depending on how much nicotine a person takes in and his or her mood at the time, the drug can act either as a stimulant or a sedative. That is why smokers may describe their first cigarette of the day as "waking them up." It also explains why a cigarette after a meal "relaxes" them.

Nicotine differs from cocaine and heroin in one important way. Most drugs, including marijuana, ecstasy, and inhalants, have an intoxicating effect. People who use such drugs become clumsy, confused, and disoriented. Nicotine does not have these effects.

In 1996, scientists at Brookhaven Laboratory, a major nuclear research facility, used body-scanning technology to discover that smokers have low levels of an **enzyme** called monoamine oxidase B (MAO B) in their brains. Enzymes trigger chemical reactions in the body, such as digesting food or breaking down body chemicals. MAO B is called the "killjoy chemical" because it breaks down dopamine, turning off feelings of pleasure in the brain.

Something in cigarette smoke stops, or *inhibits,* MAO B. Physicians use MAO inhibitors to treat people suffering from depression. It seems that smoking not only delivers nicotine to the body but also prolongs the pleasurable effects of nicotine and may even have a long-term effect on a smoker's mood.

The Brookhaven researchers made a further discovery in 2003. Comparing full-body scans of smokers and nonsmokers, they also found low levels of MAO B in the heart, liver, and kidneys of smokers. MAO B breaks down chemicals that cause high blood pressure. Since surges in blood pressure can cause crippling and even fatal strokes, this discovery points to a new health concern for smokers. Along with other recent findings, these discoveries show that there is still much more to learn about the effects smoking—and nicotine—have on the body.

Besides releasing dopamine to create feelings of pleasure, are there any positive aspects connected with nicotine? Smokers find that nicotine helps them concentrate in noisy environments. It also helps control their appetite, especially the desire for sweets. Smokers often worry that if they quit, they will gain weight. Perhaps the most important effect of nicotine on the brain is the way that it helps people handle stress. When smokers try to quit, stress becomes a big problem. Not only must they face their everyday problems but also the additional strain of breaking a powerful habit. Still worse, their usual way of dealing with difficulties—lighting up a cigarette—is now a problem in itself.

It is general knowledge that it is difficult to give up an addictive substance. Less is known about *tolerance*, the process in which a body becomes used to an addictive substance. Users have to take in ever-larger doses of the substance to feel its effects, which is why smokers increase their habits from single cigarettes to a pack a day, or even more.

Nicotine has a fairly short life span in the body. Half the amount taken in with a cigarette is gone within 40 minutes. What happens then? Many smokers light up their next cigarette.

TEENS SPEAK

I Thought One Wouldn't Hurt

Lorraine is an 18-year-old high school senior. She intends to go to college and study nursing.

"It was the summer of my sophomore year. I had just turned 16, and I was going out with a guy who smoked. Whenever he had his pack out, he offered me a cigarette. It was something he wanted us to share."

She shrugs. "Finally, I took one. I remember thinking, 'One can't hurt.'"

"I found it so strong! Couldn't even finish it. I thought I was going to faint. Bobby laughed."

Her smile at the memory fades away. "But it wasn't just one. I had more with Bobby. And I finished them, too. Finally, I was buying my own.

"I don't know when I started smoking every day. Bobby and I broke up before the Junior Prom. I was pretty upset, and the smoking seemed to help."

She holds up her pack of cigarettes. "Bobby's gone, but I always have these to remember him by. Always—that's a scary word. I've tried to quit three times, but the longest I lasted was a week.

When I did some research online, I found that lots of kids like me try to quit. Only about 3 percent make it. All because of one cigarette."

SPIKING TOBACCO

Given that nicotine is an addictive substance, do the people who provide this drug—the tobacco companies—manipulate the dose to keep smokers smoking?

In 1994, an ABC-TV newsmagazine, *Day One,* ran several stories suggesting that tobacco companies manipulated the nicotine content of cigarettes. Philip Morris, a major tobacco company, sued the network for $10 billion. Even for a large business like ABC, a $10 billion loss would be damaging. In addition, the network was in the process of being sold, and the lawsuit threatened to kill the deal. Although the news division assembled considerable evidence to back its stories, ABC executives decided to settle out of court. The TV network apologized and paid the tobacco company's legal fees.

Does that mean cigarettes are not spiked? In 1997, The Associated Press, an international news service, reported on a variety of tobacco found growing in Brazil. Called *fuomo loco* (crazy tobacco), the plants not only grow amazingly fast but also have much more nicotine than other tobacco plants. A 1998 follow-up story by UPI, another news wire service, reported that DNA Plant Technology Corp, a company working for Brown & Williamson, a large tobacco company, had created this new variety of tobacco through genetic manipulation. The company pleaded guilty to illegally exporting seeds for the plants outside the United States.

Thus, while the question of whether cigarette companies add nicotine to their products has never been proved, there is evidence that they have experimented with adding nicotine to tobacco. What else might be added?

Researchers going over tobacco company records found more than 600 ingredients added to cigarettes. Some were added for flavor, like cherry or licorice. The list included nicotine, which was described as a flavoring agent—it gives tobacco smoke its sharp, burning taste. Another chemical listed as a flavoring agent was ammonia.

It might sound strange to imagine ammonia "flavoring" anything but cleaning agents. Ammonia products are, however, used in baking dough, ice cream, pudding, and gravies. Researchers discovered that ammonia in cigarette smoke works with nicotine to create a form of the chemical that is more easily absorbed by the body. In 1996, a *Wall Street Journal* reporter revealed records from Brown & Williamson. The company's scientists had been examining a competitor's cigarettes to find out why they were so successful. Brown & Williamson researchers discovered "ammonia technology," as the process is known in the business.

The brand being analyzed was Marlboro, which had experienced a huge sales rush in the 1960s and was the best-selling brand in the world by 1979. Was its success achieved by providing Marlboro smokers a stronger nicotine kick?

Philip Morris, the company behind Marlboro, would not answer questions regarding the article, although they had earlier denied using ammonia to boost nicotine. Brown & Williamson also refused to comment on the story, claiming that its research records were a "trade secret." It also denied that ammonia increased the amount of nicotine a smoker received.

Scientists examining "ammonia technology" called it *freebasing,* a process much like the one used to create a stronger dose of cocaine. Tobacco companies continued to state that they use ammonia compounds to improve the taste of cigarettes. They also dispute the results of tests conducted by the Food and Drug Administration, the government agency responsible for the safety of foods and medicines, about the effects of adding ammonia to cigarettes.

As for references to spiking found by various antismoking activist groups and researchers in company records, the tobacco companies accuse their opponents of "cherry-picking"—taking statements out of context from thousands of documents created over a period of 40 years.

Fact Or Fiction?

I don't know what the big deal is. I can quit smoking any time I want.

The Facts: According to statistics reported by the Campaign for Tobacco-Free Kids, almost 75 percent of regular smokers in high school tried to quit but failed. Only one in seven have successfully stopped smoking for at least 30 days. Although 97 percent of high school students think they will have stopped smoking in five.years, research shows that more than 60 percent are still regular smokers after seven years.

A QUESTION THAT WON'T GO AWAY

The addictive properties of nicotine—and its other effects on the body—turn the simple act of lighting a cigarette into a health risk. In fact, there have been repeated accusations that tobacco companies manipulate the amount of nicotine in cigarettes in order to influence their addictive nature.

Q & A

Question: How do I know when I'm addicted?

Answer: Some people feel cravings for nicotine after only a few cigarettes. Others can smoke for a while without becoming addicted. Researchers say you are addicted if you answer yes to the following questions:

- Do you light up soon after you wake up in the morning?
- Do you begin to feel cravings when you are in a place where you're not allowed to smoke?
- If you were sick in bed, would you still smoke?

See also: Body and Smoking, The; Cancer and Smoking; Cardiovascular Disease and Smoking; Respiratory Diseases and Smoking; Media and Smoking, The

FURTHER READING

Goldmann, David R., ed. *American College of Physicians Complete Home Medical Guide.* New York: DK Publishing, 2003.

Hoffman, John, and Susan Froemke. *Addiction: Why Can't They Just Stop?* New York: Rodale Publishing, 2007.

Novartis Foundation. *Understanding Nicotine and Tobacco Addiction.* Hoboken, N.J.: Wiley, 2006.

■ ADVERTISING AND SMOKING

For more than 200 years, advertising—first on signs, then in newspapers and magazines, and later on radio and television—made smoking popular and tobacco companies rich. The struggle to get cigarette advertising off the air helped launch today's antismoking movement, and continuing controversies over how cigarette promotion is conducted—and who the targets are—set off some of the major arguments in tobacco control.

THE GROWTH OF TOBACCO ADVERTISING

The first recorded tobacco ad appeared in a New York newspaper in 1798 for the products of the Lorillard brothers. Founded in 1760, the Lorillard Corporation is one of the six major tobacco manufacturers today. The company made the transition from creating handmade products to mass-producing cigarettes by machine. Just as technology enabled giant growth in the tobacco industry, the development of color printing created an explosion in advertising—and explosive growth for the agencies that created advertisements. Each industry fueled the success of the other.

In 2001, *Advertising Age*, the major trade journal covering the advertising business in the United States, launched a web site that looks back at the 20th century as "The Advertising Century." The magazine listed the 100 most effective advertising campaigns. When one considers all the advertising that has been done for cars, clothes, soft drinks, and fast-food chains, it might be surprising to discover that five of the all-time best ads promoted cigarettes.

Advertising agencies often create characters portrayed by actors or even cartoons to serve as a spokesperson or symbol for a product. From Tony the Tiger telling us that Frosted Flakes are "Grrrrrrrreat!" to the Energizer Bunny going on and on, Americans encounter a vast number of characters in advertisements. Cigarette ads featured the most famous advertising figure—and also the most controversial.

The Marlboro Man is *Advertising Age's* most recognized character, a tough, strong but silent spokesman for cigarette smoking. The ad campaign started in the late 1950s, originally showing a smoker in a variety of manly occupations—lifeguard, pilot, and drill sergeant—but the public responded best to the cowboy.

Before the manly makeover, Marlboro was considered a British import that was purchased mainly by women. The ad slogan in those early days was "Marlboro—as mild as May," and print ads featured talking babies.

Marlboro's image got a complete face-lift when the brand offered a filter cigarette, capturing the interest—and brand loyalty—of many young people. A whole generation started smoking Marlboros, and many people still do. In 1950, the most successful cigarette in the United States was Camel, selling 98.2 billion packs a year. Marlboro wasn't even in the top 10. By 1970, Marlboro ranked number three, with sales of 51.37 billion packs. The brand rose to the top in 1979. Although the cigarette market was considerably smaller than it had been in the 1950s, Marlboro sold 103.6 billion packs in 1979.

The year 1979 also featured a strange contrast between image and reality at the stockholders meeting for Philip Morris, the company behind the Marlboro brand. The actor/model who had portrayed the original Marlboro Man, a smoker who was then dying of cancer, asked the company to stop their aggressive advertising. The company refused. According to *Business Week*, in 2007 the Marlboro brand ranked 14th in "The Best Global Brands 2007." This includes brands from other sectors, such as automotive, beverages, computer products, and so forth. Within the tobacco industry, it ranked number one and was worth $21.3 billion.

Camel cigarettes also have a place in advertising history. When launched in 1913, the brand revolutionized the flavor of cigarettes with a special "American Blend" of tobacco. A series of innovative advertising campaigns turned Camel into the first national brand. By 1919, 38 percent of all cigarettes made in the United States were Camels. Compared to the filtered cigarettes of the 1960s, however, Camels seemed rough. Camel smokers were older. By 1979, Camel had fallen to number seven in sales.

The company's response was to develop a filter cigarette with a taste that would attract beginning smokers—young people. Getting the attention of this young market meant introducing a new advertising campaign. Camel ads featured Joe Camel, a cartoon figure who played a saxophone, wore sunglasses and a leather jacket, and generally enjoyed doing slightly rebellious things.

Joe also offered tickets to rock concerts and "Camel Cash." Depending on the number of coupons people collected, they could acquire a wide range of items bearing Joe's picture and the Camel logo, including baseball caps, backpacks, and jackets. The merchandise was obviously aimed at young people. When the campaign was launched in 1987, only one-half of 1 percent of people under age 18 smoked Camels. By 1991, almost one-third of those age 18 had become Camel smokers.

Many adults complained that the company was targeting children. A 1991 study published in *The Journal of the American Medical Association* supported that view. It showed that more than 90 percent of the six-year-olds surveyed could identify Joe Camel, about the same percentage as those who recognized Mickey Mouse.

In response to the complaints, the company said it was not trying to get children to smoke but to ensure product identification among young people who were going to smoke anyway.

In 1997, however, R.J. Reynolds stopped using Joe Camel. They did this because of increasing legal pressures regarding the Joe Camel advertising campaign. In 1991, an attorney named Janet Mangini filed a lawsuit against R.J. Reynolds to stop using the campaign. Mangini, who practiced family law, claimed the campaign was targeted toward youth. The lawsuit gained traction when 23 state attorney generals, the American Lung Association, the American Heart Association, and the American Cancer Society all filed legal briefs supporting the lawsuit. The legal battles continued until 1997, when R.J. Reynolds decided to settle. Part of the settlement involved discontinuing the Joe Camel campaign.

TARGETING NEW SMOKERS

However one might interpret the Joe Camel controversy, it shows that tobacco companies are targeting young people. Why? In plain business terms, the tobacco companies always need new customers, especially since so many of their older customers die. The American Lung Association estimates that one million new smokers a year must be recruited for the tobacco companies to maintain their profits.

Thirty percent of smokers began at age 18. Only 5 percent of new recruits came into the habit at 24, and the percentages drop after that. In addition, smokers who start young (and some start as young as 13 or 14) offer the most profit. They spend many years smoking, and they tend to be loyal to the brands they started with, as is evident from the continuing success of Marlboro and, more recently, Camel.

Some groups are more difficult to persuade than others. Smoking among educated Caucasian males, for instance, has dropped over the years. Cigarette companies have therefore looked to other groups to recruit new smokers. One target market has been females. Since the 1920s, certain brands targeted women. The 1960s saw major new brands, like Virginia Slims, marketed to a new generation of women. Both of those eras also saw a substantial rise in the number of young women who smoked. Cigarette companies say they simply cashed in on a growing trend. In 1960, about 10 percent of cigarette ads appeared in women's magazines. By 1985, advertising had increased by 34 percent. According to a 2007 report by the Federal Trade Commission, cigarette manufacturers spent $44.8 million on magazine advertising in 2005. This is down from $95.7 million in 2004 and $156.4 million in 2003. The all-time high for spending money on magazine advertising occurred in 1984, when the industry spent $425.9 million.

Magazines for people with expensive tastes like *GQ* often have ads for cigars and some brands of cigarettes. Very different brands appear in a general-interest magazine like *Time*, or in supermarket tabloids. Edgy magazines like *Maxim,* aimed at young males, might have ads for smokeless tobacco. A magazine like *Lucky,* aimed at young women, often advertises other brands. And magazines with a predominantly black readership, like *Ebony,* will probably show ads for menthol cigarettes, which African-American smokers seem to prefer.

Tobacco companies place their ads to catch the eyes—and the taste—of potential customers. Whose eyes might they be trying to catch? Several groups have a smaller percentage of smokers than average. By targeting them, tobacco companies can recruit new smokers from previously unexploited markets. Consider this: 24.3 percent of Caucasian-American males and 19.7 percent of Caucasian-American females smoke. Only 27.6 percent of African-American women smoke versus 19.2 percent of African-American men. In the Latino community, 20.1 percent of the men and only 10.1 percent of the women smoke. Percentages of smokers among people of Asian ethnicity are even smaller.

How do the tobacco companies view the people they set out to recruit as smokers? In the BBC-TV documentary "Tobacco Wars," a former tobacco spokesperson turned antismoking crusader related a chilling comment from a major executive. Many of the people running the company didn't smoke tobacco themselves. As the executive put it, "We just reserve the right to sell it to the young, the poor, the black, the stupid."

Fact Or Fiction?

Cigarette companies don't really target young people.

The Facts: Cigarette companies need young smokers to make up for older smokers who quit or die. The earlier a smoker starts, the more profit for the tobacco companies. Check any youth-oriented magazine like *Sports Illustrated,* and you'll find cigarette ads. Check a magazine for older readers, like *Ladies' Home Journal,* and you're more likely to find advertisements for products that help smokers quit.

THE BAN

Before 1964, people smoked in offices, theaters, even in airplanes. Nearly one-half of all adult Americans enjoyed lighting up. Can you imagine an interviewer smoking a cigarette as he speaks with the world's newsmakers on television? One of TV's most respected newsmen did exactly that on a major interview show during the 1950s. Every channel ran advertisements for dozens of brands of cigarettes. Cigarette slogans and jingles were a major part of popular culture.

Then, in 1964, Surgeon General Luther Terry, the country's leading health authority, issued a report linking cigarette smoking with cancer. It resulted in a law requiring a warning on every pack of cigarettes: "Caution: Cigarette smoking may be hazardous to your health."

A second report followed in 1967. In that year, the Federal Communications Commission (FCC), the government agency overseeing broadcasting in the United States, decided to apply the Fairness Doctrine to cigarette advertising. The rule had originally been drafted to ensure that both sides of political questions would be covered. However, several activists convinced the regulators that television stations should offer time for antismoking commercials as well as for cigarette ads. By 1969, Congress was considering the idea of banning all cigarette commercials from TV and radio. Of the major networks of the day, only CBS volunteered to refuse tobacco ads. NBC and ABC rejected the notion.

In 1970, Congress passed the legislation, and the ban went into effect in 1971. The law also called for a stronger label on every pack of cigarettes: "Warning: The surgeon general has determined that cigarette smoking is dangerous to your health."

On January 2, 1971, cigarette ads disappeared from the airwaves, as did the antismoking messages required under the Fairness Doctrine. Interestingly, in the year after the antitobacco ads stopped, consumption of cigarettes rose.

THE TOBACCO INDUSTRY'S RESPONSE

Although stations could no longer broadcast advertisements, cigarette brand names and logos continued to appear on television. As early as 1968, tobacco companies were sponsoring race cars. In the 1970s, they started sponsoring entire sporting events, like Winston Cup racing (begun in 1975) and the Virginia Slims tennis tournaments (1971–94).

In 1995, the Justice Department closed another loophole that allowed tobacco companies to receive air time. Marlboro was forced to take down a number of billboards in sports arenas. The huge signs had been placed where TV cameras were most likely to be focused, such as over the players' entrances to the arena or behind the goal posts.

A fact sheet issued in 2003 by the American Lung Association points out that if you compare advertising and promotion budgets from before the ban on broadcast advertising and the present, you'd find that tobacco companies today now spend 23 times more than what they did in 1971.

Q & A

Question: My friend just switched to a low-tar, low-nicotine brand because the ads claim it's safer. Will this new brand help him to cut down and quit?

Answer: A 2004 study found people who smoke low-tar cigarettes die at the same rate as those who smoke regular varieties. If your friend really wants to stop smoking and feels the need for help, suggest that he talk to a doctor about nicotine replacement therapy.

In 2005 (the most recent year with figures available), tobacco companies spent $13.1 billion on advertising and promotion. This amount includes costs for sponsoring sporting events like the Winston Cup and cultural affairs like dance performances at New York's Lincoln Center. Advertising money exerts considerable influence on newspapers and magazines. In 1978, for instance, the *Columbia Journalism Review* examined how various publications were covering the health aspects of smoking in the seven years since the TV advertising ban. Although political, health, and legal experts continued to challenge tobacco company claims that the dangers of smoking were "not proven," not a single in-depth article appeared. Newspapers and magazines seemed unwilling to offend major advertisers.

When *Mother Jones* did a cover story on smoking in 1979, the magazine informed tobacco advertisers about the planned story as a courtesy, reasoning that they might want to withdraw their advertising for that issue. In fact, the major cigarette companies withdrew their advertising from the magazine for several years.

A POWERFUL WEAPON

Tobacco companies have used advertising to promote their products and silence criticism. Although no magazines have been punished as seriously as *Mother Jones*, major broadcasting networks like ABC and CBS have been threatened with expensive lawsuits when their newscasters prepared exposés on the tobacco industry. The companies that make up Big Tobacco won't hesitate to use financial and legal leverage to avoid damaging news stories.

See also: Media and Smoking, The

FURTHER READING
Gately, Iain. *Tobacco*. New York: Grove Press, 2002.
Haugen, David M. *How Does Advertising Impact Teen Behavior?* Farmington Hills, Mich.: Greenhaven Press, 2008.
Penncock, Angela E. *Advertising Sin and Sickness: The Politics of Alcohol and Tobacco Marketing, 1950–1990*. Dekalb: Northern Illinois Press, 2007.
Wright, R. George. *Selling Words: Free Speech in a Commercial Culture*. New York: New York University Press, 1997.

■ ALCOHOL AND TOBACCO USE

The link between drinking and smoking. An article published in 1996 in the *Journal of Addictive Diseases* underscored this link. Researchers discovered that nearly 90 percent of alcoholics were smokers. Smoking is almost three times as prevalent among alcoholics as among the general population.

TEENS SPEAK

I Tried Smoking and Then My Friends Started Drinking

Jay, a 17-year-old high school senior, played cards with a bunch of his buddies every Friday night.

"Looking back, it started as a joke, I guess. One of the guys scored a bunch of cigars, so we lit them up. It was like something out of the movies—you know, playing cards and smoking cigars.

"I liked it enough that I moved on to cigarettes. Then the beer began showing up at our card games. A big deal was to get some forties—40-ounce bottles. We wound up playing some pretty funny card games, with all sorts of crazy rules. I didn't think it was a real problem. All of us were doing it together. We only drank on weekends, so it really didn't hurt with school or anything. Besides, my crew isn't all that big on grades.

"The problem was getting the beer. Since I looked the oldest, that became my job. Really, it was no problem—'til the cops nailed me for buying beer with a fake ID. I guess our town doesn't mind teenaged smoking, but they don't like drunk driving—especially by kids.

So now I've got an arrest record. That's going to look great when I try to get a job or get into college. Not to mention that it means I already have a big strike against me if I do anything else stupid.

A DANGEROUS GATEWAY

Young people seem to discover smoking and drinking at the same time. Cigarettes and alcoholic beverages can be found in many houses. Although both substances are legal, they're the first "drugs" teenagers can get their hands on and experiment with. As a result, both are listed as "gateway drugs."

The image of a teen with a cigarette dangling from the lips and a beer can in the hand is almost a stereotype. Depending on the point of view, the label to be attached to that image can range from "edgy" or "cool" to "loser." The National Institute on Drug Abuse (NIDA) completed a 10-year study of student attitudes about alcohol and tobacco in 1986. According to that study, 18.4 percent of high school seniors who smoked also drank daily in contrast to a rate of 1.7 percent among nonsmoking seniors. Nearly 68 percent of the seniors who smoked also drank heavily, while only 17.2 percent of nonsmoking seniors engaged in heavy drinking.

In the 2006 National Survey on Drug Use and Health, researchers reported that 20.4 percent of current smokers (ages 12 and older) used illicit drugs in the past month. Two-thirds (66.3 percent) of current smokers report using alcohol in the past month. Further, 43.6 percent of current smokers report binge drinking, and 16.0 percent report heavy drinking, both in the past month. The survey also shows that 32.6 percent of heavy drinkers used illicit drugs in the past month. Only 6.4 percent of drinkers (not heavy or binge drinkers) report illicit drug use during the past month.

These statistics suggest obvious dangers, such as traffic accidents. But smoking and drinking also result in a range of less obvious dangers.

Fact Or Fiction?

Cigarettes and alcohol aren't that dangerous. After all, they're legal.

The Facts: Unlike a lot of drugs, tobacco and alcohol have been part of American culture for centuries. The fact that they've been around all that time and using them is legal doesn't mean that these drugs are safe. If alcohol and tobacco came out as products today, with their addictive properties and health risks, they would never be allowed on the market.

HEALTH CONCERNS

Counselors trying to help alcoholics have long reported that many recovering patients die young from tobacco-related diseases and conditions. More recent research expands on that observation.

A 2003 study on the effect of vitamins in protecting against cancer revealed some unexpected information. People treated for intestinal polyps, growths (sometimes cancerous) which protrude from the wall of the intestine, were offered various mixtures of beta carotene and vitamins. They were also questioned on various health matters. While most showed improvement, those who smoked and drank had a twice as high rate of polyp recurrence.

Smokers who drink regularly are twice as likely to suffer from a genetic mutation connected with lung cancer than nondrinking smokers. Scientists are just beginning to study the phenomenon. It may be that alcohol interferes with the body's systems for neutralizing and getting rid of carcinogens (cancer-causing chemicals) from cigarette smoke. Alcohol may also disrupt the body's ability to repair genes, which serve as blueprints for creating new cells in the body. Alcohol may even cause damage to genes, creating changes, or mutations, in new cells. Such changes can create cancer cells. Moderate drinking (one to two drinks a day) can increase the risk of cancer two to three times. Smoking and drinking pushes the risk to 15 times normal.

Q & A

Question: How can I talk to someone who may have a smoking and drinking problem?

Answer: Show that you're worried, not only about what the person is doing but about the direction in which they're headed. This isn't a crisis that happened overnight. Risky habits grow little by little, unnoticed by friends or even the people themselves. The problem is, they lead to bigger risks—like hard drugs, or maybe a drunk-driving accident.

Speaking up may be a wake-up call for a friend. It takes a lot of lying, cheating, and stealing for underage smokers and drinkers to get what they want. Ask your friend if that is a road he or she really wants to travel.

THE CHEMISTRY OF MIXING ALCOHOL
AND NICOTINE

Researchers are beginning to study exactly what happens when people mix alcohol and nicotine. The prevailing theory had been that people are self-medicating, using one drug to control the unwelcome effects of another. Alcohol is a sedative—it relaxes the body and brain, sometimes to the point of sleepiness. On the other hand, nicotine revs the body up—it's a stimulant. Some scientists believe that drinkers may use nicotine to wake themselves up, while smokers use alcohol to calm themselves down.

The latest research, however, seems to challenge this long-held view. In the February/March 2004 issue of *Nicotine and Tobacco Research,* investigators from Duke University showed that alcoholic drinks may enhance the pleasure provided by nicotine. The subjects were smokers who had at least four alcoholic drinks a week. Researchers first served the smokers drinks that either contained alcohol or appeared to contain alcohol but didn't and recorded how much the subjects enjoyed their cigarettes. Repeating the experiment, researchers provided some of the smokers with nicotine-free cigarettes. In a final round of experiments, some received a drug that counteracted the effects of nicotine. The results suggest that nicotine enjoyment is enhanced by even small amounts of alcohol. Subjects also reported that the experience of drinking and smoking is diminished without the nicotine.

Researchers in another study came to a similar conclusion. In a 2007 report published in *Psychopharmacology,* the authors examined social smokers who are also heavy drinkers. Social smokers are not addicted to smoking. They smoke occasionally, usually in social settings, such as parties, bars, and restaurants. The results indicated that heavy drinkers who smoke socially are more likely to smoke in social settings while drinking. The study also found that the urge to smoke gets stronger the more a person drinks. Based on their findings, the authors believe smoking enhances the stimulating properties of alcohol.

Research into this newfound relationship between the two drugs may lead to treatments that help with dependence on both nicotine and alcohol at the same time.

A PROBLEM WITH STOPPING

Visit a typical recovery program for alcoholics (people addicted to alcohol)—Alcoholics Anonymous, for example—and you'll find a group of heavy smokers huddled in the back seats or catching a quick smoke outside. When alcoholics try to stop drinking, they often smoke heavily to keep from relapsing.

As those who have helped alcoholics recover have noted, this often means that many recovering alcoholics die from smoking-related diseases rather than alcohol-related ones. For instance, both founders of Alcoholics Anonymous died of lung cancer.

People who have quit smoking often relapse when they drink. Researchers have also discovered that people with an alcohol problem, even a past alcohol problem, have greater difficulty in quitting smoking. From the beginning of the recovery movement in the 1950s, however, the general wisdom was "you can only quit one thing at a time."

As evidence of the addictive aspects of tobacco has grown, people working in the fields of substance abuse and mental health treatment are finding it more and more difficult to allow patients merely to switch addictions. As medical research reveals more about the interaction of nicotine and alcohol in the brain, treatment specialists may be able to develop relief for both dependencies.

See also: Drugs and Tobacco Use

FURTHER READING

Alters, Sandra M. *Alcohol, Tobacco, and Illicit Drugs.* Farmington, Mich.: Information Plus Reference Series, 2007.

Brizer, David. *Quitting Smoking for Dummies.* New York: Wiley, 2003.

Hoffman, John, and Susan Froemke. *Addiction: Why Can't They Just Stop?* New York: Rodale Publishing, 2007.

▨ ANTISMOKING ADVOCACY GROUPS

Organizations opposed to the tobacco industry and smoking. Antismoking advocacy groups have waged a "war" on the tobacco industry. The goals of these groups are to educate the public on the dangers of tobacco, help people stop smoking, prevent youth from taking up the habit, and expose the lies that tobacco companies have often used to sell cigarettes and other tobacco products.

Although antismoking advocates have been part of our society for more than 400 years, active antismoking advocacy in the United States really took off after the 1964 report by the Surgeon General. The report conclusively identified a link between smoking and illnesses. Since that time, the tobacco industry has been under fire by government agencies, health associations, and advocacy groups.

BRIEF HISTORY OF ANTISMOKING ADVOCACY

Antismoking advocacy is not new. Smoking bans have been used for centuries. During the 1600s, Pope Urban VIII banned smoking in holy places. Leaders of many countries, such as China, Russia, Italy, Japan, and England, have had various restrictions and bans on smoking. During early colonial times, there were also smoking restrictions and bans. For example, in Connecticut, residents were allowed to smoke only once a day. The act of smoking had to occur in a private place, as public smoking was strictly prohibited. As time went on, the tobacco trade become very profitable. Eventually, bans around the world were lifted so governments could profit as well.

In the 1964 report, the Surgeon General discussed the relationship between smoking and health. In particular, he noted that there is a clear relationship between smoking and lung cancer in both men and women. The Surgeon General estimated that smokers were approximately 10 times more likely to develop lung cancer than nonsmokers. The latest estimate from the Centers for Disease Control and Prevention (CDC) indicates that men who smoke are 22 times more likely than nonsmokers to die from lung cancer. The CDC estimates that women smokers are now 12 times more likely than women nonsmokers to die from lung cancer.

Since the 1964 Surgeon General's report, the tobacco industry has been faced with increasing bans and restrictions. Laws have been passed banning television advertisements for cigarettes, smoking on airplanes and buses, and smoking in public places—including bars and restaurants.

Probably the biggest blow to the tobacco industry came in 1998 with the signing of the Master Settlement Agreement (MSA). Tobacco companies were faced with lawsuits by most states. The states wanted to get back money they had spent on treating smoking-related illnesses through Medicaid and Medicare. The MSA was an agreement between four tobacco companies (Brown & Williamson Tobacco Corporation, Lorillard Tobacco Company, Philip Morris Incorporated, R.J. Reynolds

Tobacco Company) and 46 states plus five U.S. territories. (The remaining four states settled their lawsuits separately.) As part of the settlement, tobacco companies pay the states several hundred-million dollars per year. From a public relations standpoint, the most damaging aspect of the settlement was the release of confidential industry documents. Among other things, the documents included research findings on the addictiveness of tobacco, marketing strategies designed to get children to smoke, and some of the health consequences of smoking. These documents have provided antismoking groups with plenty of ammunition to use attacking the tobacco industry.

Fact Or Fiction?

The antismoking advocacy groups are not working in the best interest of the public.

The Facts: Antismoking advocacy groups are working to prevent smoking, help smokers quit, expose the tobacco industry's manipulative marketing techniques, and reduce exposure to secondhand smoke. From a health standpoint, the groups are working in the public's best interest. From a civil liberties perspective, many feel the advocacy groups are going too far and infringing on the individual freedoms. In particular, bans on smoking in public places, restaurants, and bars is seen as being too excessive. Ultimately, however, you have to decide whether these groups are working for the best interest of both the public and you.

TYPES OF ADVOCACY GROUPS

Several types of advocacy groups exist. They range from government-sponsored groups to associations and societies to private groups that are on a crusade to inform the public about smoking and end the tobacco industry.

Agencies within both federal and state governments position themselves as against smoking. These include Departments of Health, Centers for Disease Control, and several institutes within the National Institutes of Health. The CDC's Office of Smoking and Health is considered the government's primary agency for tobacco control.

Federal and state agencies all warn against the dangers of smoking. They produce literature designed to educate consumers. This includes data on the prevalence of smoking, the financial costs of smoking, and smoking-related diseases. These agencies advocate antismoking legislation designed to create smoke-free workplaces, reduce smoking in public places, and impose tougher laws to prevent teenagers from buying cigarettes. State and federal legislatures have increased cigarette taxes in the hope of reducing smoking, and this has, in general, met with success. The number of smokers drops when there are cigarette-tax increases. Higher costs also mean fewer people will be tempted to start smoking.

Health-care associations are also advocates against smoking. Associations include the American Medical Association, the American Heart Association, the American Lung Association, the American Cancer Association, the American Dental Association, and the American Diabetes Association. Canadian and European health associations also advocate against smoking. Each association focuses on the effect smoking has on their area of specialty. For example, the American Heart Association informs the public of the dangers smoking has on heart health.

Then there are the organizations that focus solely on antismoking issues. These groups are not part of government agencies or professional associations. Some of the prominent antismoking advocacy groups include ASH (Action on Smoking and Health), American Legacy Foundation, Americans for Nonsmokers' Rights, and the Campaign for Tobacco-Free Kids.

American Legacy Foundation

The American Legacy Foundation was a result of the 1998 Master Settlement Agreement (MSA), which was initially funded as part of the MSA. That funding, however, ended in 2003, and the American Legacy Foundation now relies on investments and other sources of income.

Although many people may not be familiar with the American Legacy Foundation, people will be familiar with their work. The American Legacy Foundation is responsible for the truth® campaign. The campaign delivers provocative messages about the dangers of smoking. These commercials prompted one tobacco company, Lorillard Tobacco Company, to file a lawsuit against the American Legacy Foundation. The lawsuit claimed that the truth® ads personally attack and vilify tobacco companies. In 2006, the Delaware Supreme Court ruled against Lorillard, saying the ads do not qualify as personal attacks or vilifications of tobacco companies.

Action on Smoking and Health

Action on Smoking and Health (ASH) is another large nonprofit advocacy group. ASH has chapters across the world, notably in Britain and Australia. ASH advocates for nonsmokers' rights and plays a role in legal actions concerning smoking. The organization also acts as an information clearinghouse on smoking related-issues. The ASH Web sites provide information on smoking, policy issues, lawsuits, and the latest smoking-related news.

Americans for Nonsmokers' Rights

Americans for Nonsmoker's Rights (ANR) bills itself as the leading national lobby for nonsmokers' rights. Their goal is similar to other groups': reduce and prevent tobacco addiction among juveniles and protect nonsmokers from exposure to secondhand smoke. The last goal is their area of specialty. The ANR helps localities pass smoke-free ordinances. The organization has been recognized by the U.S. Surgeon General as the leader in the field of clean indoor-air policy.

Campaign for Tobacco-Free Kids

The Campaign for Tobacco-Free Kids works to change public policies and attitudes about smoking. It seeks to prevent juveniles from smoking, protect nonsmokers from secondhand smoke, and help smokers overcome their addiction. The campaign is very active and has been deemed "the country's leading anti-tobacco lobby" by the *New York Times.*

The campaign has played an important role in helping states secure funding for tobacco-prevention programs. It works with other advocates to help increase the amount of money states spend on tobacco-control programs.

Another initiative has been to work with public health organizations to convince the U.S. Congress to grant the Food and Drug Administration (FDA) regulatory authority over tobacco. Right now, the FDA does not have this authority.

THE TRUTH®

One of the most popular antismoking campaigns is the truth® from the American Legacy Foundation. The campaign was started in 2000 and is considered the largest national youth smoking-prevention campaign.

The goal of the campaign is to counter advertising by the tobacco industry. To reach youth, the truth® campaign designs thought-provoking messages. For example, one commercial shows members of the truth® driving supply trucks to the front of a corporate tobacco office in a large city. Then they dump 1,200 body bags on the street, representing the estimated 1,200 who people die from smoking each day.

Another commercial shows members of the truth® entering a smoking convention to give away samples of "Ammoniade." The commercial is based on the fact that ammonia is added to cigarettes. Internal tobacco documents indicate that ammonia is used to increase the amount of freebase nicotine, which increases addiction. Tobacco companies, however, argue that ammonia is used to enhance flavor. Thus, using that same logic, the truth® squad wants to give out free samples of "Ammoniade" because it tastes so good.

Q & A

Question: Do antismoking campaigns work?

Answer: Research indicates that antismoking campaigns do work. The American Legacy Foundation conducted research to see if the truth® campaigns are effective. The results show that 75 percent of youth, ages 12–17, can recall at least one truth® commercial. The results also reveal that the truth® campaigns are responsible for approximately 22 percent of the decline in youth smoking between 1999 and 2002.

In a 2005 study in *Tobacco Control*, researchers found that television advertisements were effective in getting smokers to call a national quit-smoking hotline. Similar findings occurred in a 2006 study in the *American Journal of Preventative Medicine*. The authors of that study found that former smokers most frequently cited antitobacco advertisements as a source of help.

FURTHER READING

Chapman, Simon. *Public Health Advocacy and Tobacco Control: Making Smoking History*. New York: Wiley-Blackwell, 2007.

■ BODY AND SMOKING, THE

To communicate, the various systems of the body rely on a great variety of chemical messengers. **Hormones** are chemicals that control local organ functions or that initiate or inhibit bodywide responses. **Cytokines** are chemicals that activate or suppress the immune system, the body's defenses against bacteria and viruses. **Neurotransmitters** are chemicals that help transmit impulses across the spaces between nerve cells or between nerve and muscle cells.

In addition to these messengers, there are **enzymes**, chemicals that turn on and off chemical reactions such as digesting various elements in food or breaking down chemicals to be excreted. With hormones, cytokines, neurotransmitters, and enzymes, the average body is a complex chemical stew. Smoking adds thousands of random chemicals to this mixture. The best-known chemical in the new mix is nicotine, which has serious effects on the brain. But nicotine also affects systems in the other parts of the body. Tobacco smoke contains other chemicals that can have serious effects on body organs as well.

TEENS SPEAK

Smoking Changes You

Erin is a lively 17-year-old high school senior. She has never smoked, and is a founding member of REBEL—Reaching Everyone By Exposing Lies, a New Jersey antismoking activist group.

"Our first slogan was 'not for sale.' We just decided we weren't going to give in to the manipulation and lies. Why would you take years off your life because of an advertisement? It's like the tobacco companies are putting a price on our heads."

She leans forward. "That's our driving reason. Our second slogan is 'My mind, my body, my choice.' You see people putting all those toxins into their bodies, stuff that isn't supposed to be in there, and doing it in mass quantities. It throws everything out of whack.

"We knew some of the facts already. But the Surgeon General's latest report on smoking shows that it's not just bad for one or two parts of the body, it's bad for the whole system."

She grins. "And when he came out with the report, he also had some nice things to say about what we're doing in New Jersey."

Erin turns serious again. "We have to get off the cycle of having people die too young. The older generation has started dying off already. If it's going to stop, it will have to be youth—us—that does it."

NICOTINE

Nicotine stimulates brain cells to create feelings of pleasure. It also "revs up" the body, spurring the production of epinephrine from the adrenal glands. This primes the body for the **"fight or flight" response**. When our prehistoric ancestors faced danger—like a wolf or a lion, for instance, they had to be able to run for their lives or to fight desperately. Today this reaction is reserved more for unpleasant surprises—a pop quiz or having to speak in class. It can also be associated with good things, like going out for a special evening with a special person.

Whatever the reason, the results are the same. The hormone epinephrine (also known as adrenaline) sends chemical messages throughout the body. The heart speeds up by 10 to 20 beats a minute. Blood vessels constrict—that is, they get tighter. This constriction pushes blood pressure up five to 10 points. So, the heart works harder, pushing blood through narrower veins and arteries, an additional workload for a very important organ.

After 30 to 40 minutes, the effect of the nicotine starts to wear off, and the smoker begins to feel tired and depressed. The usual response is to light up another cigarette, and the cycle begins all over again. This continuous, intermittent strain on the heart and blood vessels goes on every day the smoker continues with the habit.

TAR

When someone blows a cloud of white smoke on a movie screen, it may look cool, or even pretty. In the real world, if someone blows smoke through a tissue, it leaves a yellowish–brown stain from something known as tar.

The word **tar** may bring to mind the sticky black substance used to surface streets. Like that tar, the tiny particles in cigarette smoke melt in the 2,000-degree heat near the tip of a lit cigarette. Those particles then carry nicotine into the lungs, where it enters the bloodstream. What happens to the tar? It turns solid in the lungs, getting stuck in the machinery of one of the body's most amazing systems—the **pulmonary system.**

Each time you inhale, you take in the oxygen that is needed to run every cell in your body. Every time you exhale, you get rid of the body's waste gas, carbon dioxide, in much the way the tailpipe of a car vents exhaust fumes. Unlike a car, your body manages to do both jobs with one system. Each breath brings air in through the mouth and nose. The air travels down a large tube known as the **bronchial passage**, which breaks off like the branches of a tree into ever-tinier airways. These passages lead to about three million tiny, thin-walled sacs, the **alveoli.** The walls of the alveoli are only one cell thick. Oxygen passes through this very thin tissue and enters hair-thin blood vessels, where it binds with red blood cells. Carbon dioxide passes out of the liquid part of the blood, the plasma, transferring through the alveoli walls, and is then expelled from the lungs.

The size of your lungs depends on the size of your body. Your two fists joined together are about the size of one lung. Healthy lungs are packed with an amazing 100 square yards of the thin tissues that make up the walls of the alveoli.

The lungs have several lines of defense against unwelcome substances. Mucous membranes, which line the passages to the lungs, secrete a sticky substance, mucus, to trap foreign particles and germs. Tiny hairlike structures, cilia, also grow from the walls of the air passages. The job of the cilia is to push foreign substances away from the lungs and back to the bronchial tubes, where they will be coughed up.

Unfortunately, something in cigarette smoke paralyzes the cilia. Tar particles and mucus gather in the air passages, blocking the path of oxygen. These sticky blockages are the beginnings of smoker's cough—when a smoker is constantly hacking up the debris from cigarette smoke.

Tar particles are so tiny, they can invade even the smallest alveoli. Once they're in place, they tend to stay. When doctors examine healthy lung tissue, they'll find some dirty spots. Like it or not, pollution is in the air no matter where you live. Everyone ends up breathing car exhaust and smoke particles from factories and power plants.

A smoker's lungs, however, show black specks all over, like a piece of fresh meat with a very heavy sprinkling of black pepper.

Those black specks physically block the exchange of gases in the alveoli. With mucus, they hinder the movement of air in and out of the lungs and cause chronic bronchitis, inflammation, and infection of the air passages. Worse, chemicals in tar irritate and damage the delicate lung tissues. That damage can turn into cancer.

Fact Or Fiction?

My grandfather smoked all his life, and he lived to be 90.

The Facts: Some smokers live to age 85 and older—you can see that in the statistics. The problem is that most smokers don't live that long. Be glad to have a 90-year-old smoker around. But it might be instructive to ask him what happened to all the smoking buddies he had when he was 20 years old.

CARBON MONOXIDE

Starting from the lungs, blood travels through the body delivering oxygen, exchanging it with carbon dioxide, and then returning to the lungs to remove waste gases from the body. It's a system that has developed over millions of years—oxygen in, carbon dioxide out. Smoking delivers another gas into the body, messing up this long-running success story.

Carbon monoxide is a gas that is similar to carbon dioxide. Like carbon dioxide, it is odorless and colorless. Like carbon dioxide, it is also created by combustion—whether in a car engine, a fire, or the tip of a cigarette. In high enough quantities, both carbon dioxide and carbon monoxide are poisonous.

If you could magnify these incredibly small gas molecules, you would find that carbon monoxide has one oxygen atom bound to a carbon atom, while carbon dioxide has two. That tiny difference has a huge impact on the way the two gases act in the human body.

When the heart-lung system is working correctly, oxygen binds to **hemoglobin**, a chemical in red blood cells, and travels through the body to help cells create energy. Carbon dioxide dissolves into the liquid part of the blood, the **plasma**. Earth's atmosphere usually contains 210,000 parts per million of oxygen, 600 parts per million of carbon dioxide, and only 0.2 parts per million of carbon monoxide.

However, when a smoker breathes in cigarette smoke, the fraction of carbon monoxide is more like 500 to 1,500 parts per million. Once inside the lungs, carbon monoxide begins to disrupt the breathing system. The problem is, carbon monoxide molecules bind better to hemoglobin than oxygen. The poison gas molecules push oxygen out of the way. So, while tar blocks the flow of air through the lungs, carbon monoxide cuts down the amount of oxygen that reaches the bloodstream. The heart must work harder to get more blood moving through the lungs to make up for the missing oxygen. The result is an additional strain on both organs, as well as a decrease in the oxygen supply to the heart and brain. For healthy people, the amount of carbon monoxide in cigarette smoke can cause headaches and flu-like symptoms. For people who already have heart disease, carbon monoxide exposure can cause chest pains.

Q & A

Question: I've been smoking for a while now, and I'm getting a little worried. Even if I quit, will things really get better inside my body?

Answer: Getting better is a prime reason to stop smoking. The day after you quit, your chances of having a heart attack drop.

Within the first nine months after quitting, your smoker's cough should disappear and you'll find yourself not getting out of breath so quickly during physical exertion. Your lungs will be cleaner and better able to resist infections.

A year after you quit, your chances of having a heart attack are cut in half. In five years, your risk of having a stroke is the same as that of a nonsmoker. In 10 years, your chance of lung cancer is half of what it would be if you had continued smoking. In 15 years, your risk of heart disease will be the same as that of a nonsmoker.

See also: Cancer and Smoking; Cardiovascular Disease and Smoking; Respiratory Diseases and Smoking

FURTHER READING
Goldmann, David R., ed. *American College of Physicians Complete Home Medical Guide*. New York: DK Publishing, 2003.
Hyde, Margaret O., and John F. Setevo, M.P. *Smoking 101: An Overview for Teens*. Minneapolis, Minn.: Twenty-first Century Books, 2006.

■ CANCER AND SMOKING

As cancer cells multiply, they form damaging growths and can spread to other sites in the body. Cancer may be caused by a virus, radiation, sunlight, or chemicals. Cigarette smoke contains a number of cancer-causing chemicals. According to the surgeon general, the country's leading health authority, smoking is the leading cause of cancer deaths.

DNA contains the blueprint for cells and all living things, also known as the **genetic** code. Genes carry traits from parents to children. Height, looks, even hair color all come from the mixture of genes contributed by parents. Genes also determine the interior structure of the body. They ensure that organs grow in the proper places and reach the correct size. As a person grows up, oncogenes in the nucleus of tissue cells control how often those cells divide. The plan is to create only enough tissue cells to replace those that die. Sometimes genes are damaged, either by radiation or by a variety of chemicals called **carcinogens**. Oncogenes repair this damage, or if the damage can't be fixed, they program the cell to self-destruct. Sometimes, however, these mutated cells survive. They become abnormal, reproduce uncontrollably, and cancer begins. Some oncogenes are more effective than others. For people with less effective oncogenes, cancer can be seen to run in their families.

When a cell becomes abnormal, it begins to reproduce. The cell doubles, and those two cells double, the resulting four cells double, and so on. After 25 to 30 doublings, the clump of cancerous cells has become a mass approximately half an inch wide, containing billions of cells.

This growth is called a **tumor,** and it continues to get larger, invading and damaging healthy tissues around it. Cancers are named for the parts of the body where they originate, and they can damage important organs like the lungs, stomach, or brain. This damage can become fatal.

Cancer cells can also invade the blood vessels or the lymph system, part of the body's defenses against outside organisms. Cells can break off from the primary tumor and travel the blood and lymph systems like highways, creating new tumors in other parts of the body. This is called **metastasis**. If left untreated or treated too late, cancer may have spread to attack too many important organs. The patient then faces a painful, lingering death.

Although medical writers had commented on the apparent connection between smoking and cancer for centuries, serious study of the link began in the late 1920s. The general public became aware of the connection in the 1950s, as scientists began identifying cancer-causing chemicals and then discovering them in cigarette smoke. A 1989 surgeon general's report found at least 43 carcinogens in cigarette smoke.

TEENS SPEAK

It's Enough to Make You Sick

Noreen quit school at age 17. She'd been smoking for two years by that time. Presently, she works at a small restaurant. At the end of a shift, her uniform smells strongly of tobacco smoke.

"I left school because I wasn't going anywhere. Not that I'm going anywhere right now. The pay is lousy and the tips aren't great. As for benefits—ha! Not in this dump.

"Let me tell you, restaurants and bars are nothing at all like you see on TV. The kitchen stinks from fried food, and out in the dining room everybody's smoking up a storm. When I come in to start my shift, they're trying to air the place out. All you can smell is beer and old cigarettes. Then all you smell is new cigarette smoke—clouds of it.

"Half the time I'm stressed out from customers, or the boss is on me for something. I smoke every break I get, then it's back to the clouds in the restaurant. Some days I think I spend my whole shift breathing smoke. I'm starting to get this cough that's scaring me. If I get something like cancer, how can I expect to pay for it? My savings account is barely over the bank's minimum. And I have no insurance."

THE SMOKING GUN: THE NUMBERS

As early as 1602, an English writer commented on the soot-related diseases of chimney sweeps and wondered if smoking tobacco had the same effects. Over the next 200 years, some doctors noted that pipe smokers got cancer of the mouth and snuff takers got cancer of the nose. Also in the 1700s, lung cancer was discovered—a very rare disease. In 1900, lung cancer was still rare. But as the century progressed, more and more people began developing this form of cancer. It grew five times faster than any other cancer between 1938 and 1948. Today, lung cancer is the number one cancer in the world, especially in poorer, less-developed countries. It's the second most widespread cancer among American men and women and the most deadly.

Studying death statistics from 1997 to 2001, the Centers for Disease Control and Prevention (CDC) found that smoking killed over 438,000 people a year—roughly one out of every five deaths in the United States. Lung cancer and about a dozen other types of cancers accounted for over 251,000 of those deaths. The CDC concluded that cigarette smoking is the most important source of preventable illness and premature death in the world today.

THE RISKS

As they light up their first cigarettes, most young smokers aren't thinking of the consequences of smoking, but there are consequences. In terms of life expectancy, male smokers lose about 13 years off their lives. Females lose 14.5 years.

The threat of cancer plays a big part in shortening smokers' lives. Lung cancer is an obvious danger. Smokers are 10 times more likely to develop this disease than nonsmokers. But smokers have an equally large chance of developing varieties of cancer that attack the mouth and tongue, nasal passages, gums, throat, voice box, or esophagus. The risk of bladder cancer is two to three times higher for smokers than for nonsmokers. Smoking also doubles the risk of stomach cancers. In addition, smokers also are more likely to develop cancer in the kidney, pancreas, liver, cervix, colon, and rectum than nonsmokers. Smokers are at greater risk for some forms of leukemia as well.

Fact Or Fiction?

There's still a lot of controversy over cigarettes and cancer.

The Facts: If anyone still doubts that smoking causes cancer, they haven't been paying much attention to medical news for the last few years. Even the tobacco companies, who fought the hardest to dispute the connection, have had to admit the fact that their product kills people.

CHRONIC V. ACUTE CANCER

Medical people describe diseases as either **chronic** or **acute**. An acute disease is one that has a sudden onset and lasts a short time. The word *chronic* comes from the Greek word for time. A chronic disease recurs or progresses over time. A chronic cough, for instance, is one that does not go away. Cancer is usually considered chronic, progressing through certain set stages over a period of time. A lump, a sore, or a cough that won't go away may be an early sign of cancer. The earlier cancer is detected, the sooner treatment can begin.

The usual treatment for cancer is surgery to remove the tumor. For those with lung cancer, for instance, doctors may remove a portion of the lung or the entire organ. In cases where the tumor has **metastasized**, **chemotherapy** or **radiation therapy** may be used. In chemotherapy, patients receive powerful drugs to destroy fast-growing cancer cells. In radiation therapy, beams of X-rays, electrons, or gamma rays are used to destroy cancerous cells, or radioactive materials are placed in or around the tumor. Both chemotherapy and radiation affect healthy cells as well. Patients may suffer pain, vomiting, weakness, and hair loss.

Cure rates for some cancers can be as high as nine cases out of 10. In other varieties, the cure rate is more like one out of 10. If all symptoms of cancer disappear and there is no evidence of cancer cells in the body, the patient is said to be in **remission**. If the patient manages to survive for five years without the cancer returning, there is a good chance that he or she has been cured.

Acute diseases appear suddenly with a severe intensity. In acute appendicitis, sudden pain warns the patient that the organ is inflamed and in danger of bursting. In acute cancer, the onset of the disease is sudden and its progress rapid. Prompt, aggressive treatment may be required if the patient is to survive.

In either its chronic or acute forms, cancer draws away the patient's energy and causes considerable pain. Especially in the end stages, patients may receive heavy pain medication.

Q & A

Question: My dad smoked for years, and now he's sick. His doctor is talking about cancer. How do I handle this?

Answer: You'll have to learn as much as possible about your father's illness, and then figure out how you can help him and the other members of your family.

With many varieties of cancer, treatments offer patients excellent possibilities of recovery, especially if the disease was caught early. If your dad has a chance of recovering, be grateful and as helpful as possible. You may want to work with him on a plan to stop smoking. If the future looks more grim, you'll have to work through it, day by day.

Situations like these are the real test of a family. Family members either pull together or fall apart. You'll want to do your best to make sure your family is still standing, however things turn out.

See also: Body and Smoking, The; Cardiovascular Disease and Smoking; Respiratory Diseases and Smoking

FURTHER READING

Abrams, David B., Raymond Niaura, Richard A. Brown, Karen M. Emmons, Michael G. Goldstein, Peter N. Nonti, and Laura A. Linnan. *The Tobacco Dependence Treatment Handbook: A Guide to Best Practices.* New York: Guilford Press, 2003.

Goldmann, David R., ed. *American College of Physicians Complete Home Medical Guide.* New York: DK Publishing, 1999.

Springhouse. *Professional Guide to Diseases, 9th Edition.* New York: Lippincott Williams & Wilkins, 2008.

■ CARDIOVASCULAR DISEASE AND SMOKING

Some cardiovascular diseases, like heart attacks and **strokes,** can be fatal or leave patients seriously disabled. Cigarette smoke contains a number of chemicals that have been shown to damage the heart and blood vessels, setting the stage for serious, even fatal illnesses.

While pumping blood throughout the body, the **cardiovascular system** performs several functions. Blood vessels deliver oxygen and nutrients to every cell in the body, while removing carbon dioxide and wastes. The heart stays on the job 24 hours a day, seven days a week, moving the blood supply, about 10.5 pints, through the entire body about once a minute.

The blood vessels make up a complicated network that reaches every cell in the body. Laid end to end, these sections of "body plumbing" would reach almost 100,000 miles for a typical adult. Most of that distance comes from the microscopic **capillaries**, tiny blood vessels whose walls are only one cell thick. Blood leaves the heart through the arteries, the largest of which, the aorta, is about the size of a garden hose. The arteries branch off into smaller vessels, the arterioles, and then into the capillaries. These thin-walled blood vessels allow oxygen and nutrients to transfer out to the cells of the body. Waste products and carbon dioxide filter back in. The capillaries grow together into venuoles and then into veins, which head back to the heart. Blood also flows to the lungs to eliminate carbon dioxide and get a new supply of oxygen, through the digestive system for nutrients, and to the liver and kidneys where wastes are removed.

The cardiovascular system is complicated and performs a critical function. If the flow of blood becomes blocked because of disease, the results can be very serious. Several components of cigarette smoke damage blood vessels, creating the potential for cardiovascular disease, while also putting additional strain on the heart.

Fact Or Fiction?

You've got to be really old before you need to worry about the effects of smoking.

The Facts: While heart disease usually strikes older people, smoking accelerates the onset of the disease. Instead of being struck in their 70s, smokers get heart attacks in their 60s— or even in their 50s.

If those ages still seem comfortably far away, consider the short-term effects of smoking: bad breath, stained teeth, and shortness of breath impairing sports performance. Consider, too, that smokers are constantly coughing, irritating their lungs, and irritating the lungs of the people around them with cigarette smoke. Finally, add up the costs of buying a pack of cigarettes each day for a year.

CARDIOVASCULAR DISEASES

According to 2008 figures from the Centers for Disease Control and Prevention (CDC), cardiovascular diseases are responsible for nearly 35 percent of deaths every year in the United States. Approximately 870,000 Americans die of cardiovascular disease every year. The American Heart Association estimates that more than 135,000 deaths are due to smoking-related cardiovascular diseases.

Every time a smoker lights a new cigarette, the fresh dose of nicotine puts additional stress on the cardiovascular system. Nicotine pushes the heart to work faster—10 to 20 more beats per minute. Nicotine also causes the blood vessels to constrict, pushing up blood pressure five to 10 points. These are merely short-term effects of cigarette smoke. The long-term effects of smoking cause even more serious problems for the cardiovascular system.

Atherosclerosis

Smoking has been connected with **atherosclerosis**—a condition also known as hardening of the arteries. Arteries are actually complex structures, constructed to be strong and flexible. They must withstand the rush of freshly pumped blood. (In comparison, blood pressure in the veins is only one-tenth of what the arteries must handle.) Arteries must also be able to expand or close down. To meet these needs, artery walls are composed of alternating layers of expandable tissue and muscle cells.

Sometimes the innermost layer of the artery becomes damaged. The artery wall thickens as fatty deposits gather. As these **plaques** or thickened sections grow, the arteries become less elastic. The growth of plaques narrows the inside of the artery. Plaques can also break, creating blood clots which completely block an artery.

Medical researchers are still trying to understand exactly what causes atherosclerosis. They've discovered several factors, including obesity, high cholesterol, and lack of exercise. A major contributor seems to be smoking. When the arteries of smokers are compared to those of nonsmokers, smokers have less flexibility in the blood vessels and larger plaque deposits. Smoking seems to accelerate the process of hardening of the arteries.

Smokers have problems with their blood as well. The carbon monoxide in cigarette smoke binds with red blood cells, cutting down the amount of oxygen the blood can carry. Chemicals in cigarette smoke also make the blood thicker, more likely to clot. When a person cuts himself or herself, clotting is a good thing. A blood clot inside the body, however, can be dangerous.

If a blood clot catches where plaques have already partially blocked a blood vessel, it can further reduce blood flow or cut it off altogether. Blood may not reach the legs, causing weakness and pain. If blood does not reach the kidneys, the result may be a build-up of poisons in the body. A clot can even cut off the blood supply to the heart muscles—causing a heart attack.

In recent years, medical researchers have investigated the connection between inflammation and atherosclerosis. You've probably seen your skin become hot and swollen—inflamed—as a result of an infection or an allergy. Inflammation can affect many tissues, including the walls of blood vessels. It can also cause chemicals connected with clotting to appear in the blood. Scientists are trying to determine whether some of the chemicals from tobacco smoke irritate the lining of arteries, creating a recurring inflammation that weakens the artery wall. Thicker blood and higher blood pressure can then cause damage in the weakened artery wall, creating a site where a plaque may develop.

Whatever the exact cause, smoking speeds the progress of atherosclerosis. Its contribution to the disease can be fatal—especially if blockages form in the arteries feeding the heart. Damage to heart muscles can disrupt the function of the organ. The CDC estimates that nearly 82,000 people die from smoking-related heart attacks each year.

Q & A

Question: My best friend's mother—a smoker—collapsed while she was out shopping. Although they rushed her to the hospital, she died! My friend keeps going on about how her mom "dropped dead." Her own smoking has gotten very heavy all of a sudden. What can I do to help her?

Answer: One of the most devastating things about cardiovascular diseases is that they can strike with very little warning and fatal results. If your friend's mother had been ill for a while, there would have been some time to prepare. As it is, your friend is obviously dealing with a terrible shock. Smoking may be one of the ways she's handling stress.

You'll have to try and console your friend through this bad time. Help her in any way you can, especially in terms of her health. Try to make sure she gets help from other friends, adults, her religious leaders, and if necessary, from professionals.

Stroke

If an artery supplying blood to the heart muscles becomes blocked, that obstruction can cause a fatal heart attack. Smokers suffer from other blockages, too. According to Action on Smoking and Health (ASH), an antismoking group, smokers are 16 times more likely than nonsmokers to experience obstructed blood vessels in the legs and feet. Overall, smokers are 1.5 times as likely to suffer a stroke.

A stroke or cerebral thrombosis occurs when a blocked artery cuts off the flow of blood to the brain.

A stroke is sometimes called a brain attack. As with a heart attack, quick medical attention can make a difference in survival. When blood is cut off to the brain, none of the cells receive nourishment or oxygen, thus killing brain cells. Depending on which part of the brain is damaged, results can include blurry vision, memory loss, speech problems, a sudden droop in the muscles on one side of the face, weakness or inability to move one's arm or leg (or both), and paralysis of half the body. Heavy smokers (people who smoke 20 or more cigarettes a day) are two to four times more likely to suffer a stroke in their lifetimes.

If a stroke is diagnosed and treated quickly, the patient stands an improved chance of recovery. Drugs are used to dissolve the blood clot in the brain and may also be used to thin the blood so that it will flow more easily through constricted arteries. Efforts will also be made to reduce high blood pressure, which often accompanies a stroke. There will also be **rehabilitation**—speech therapy or physical therapy.

Approximately one-third of stroke victims make a full or nearly full recovery. Another one-third may be disabled to some extent, sometimes requiring help in a nursing facility. For those whose symptoms continue for six months to a year, the problem is likely to be permanent. They end up unable to move, eat, or speak normally. About 20 percent of stroke victims die in the hospital within a month of the attack. Among those deaths are more than 17,000 smokers.

AVOIDING CARDIOVASCULAR DISEASE

People can take many measures to avoid the danger of heart attack or stroke. Controlling cholesterol and blood pressure, losing weight, and adopting a more active lifestyle can all help to reduce the risk of cardiovascular disease. Smokers can remove a major risk factor by

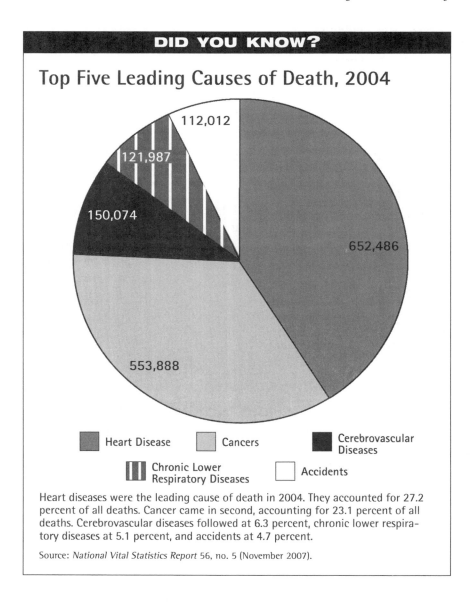

DID YOU KNOW?

Top Five Leading Causes of Death, 2004

112,012

121,987

150,074

652,486

553,888

■ Heart Disease   ■ Cancers   ■ Cerebrovascular Diseases

▥ Chronic Lower Respiratory Diseases   ☐ Accidents

Heart diseases were the leading cause of death in 2004. They accounted for 27.2 percent of all deaths. Cancer came in second, accounting for 23.1 percent of all deaths. Cerebrovascular diseases followed at 6.3 percent, chronic lower respiratory diseases at 5.1 percent, and accidents at 4.7 percent.

Source: *National Vital Statistics Report* 56, no. 5 (November 2007).

quitting the habit. As the American Cancer Society's guide to quitting points out, a smoker's risk of heart attack drops measurably just one day after quitting. The more years a smoker remains smoke-free, the lower the cardiovascular risks become.

See also: Body and Smoking, The; Cancer and Smoking; Respiratory Diseases and Smoking

FURTHER READING
Goldmann, David R., ed. *American College of Physicians Complete Home Medical Guide.* New York: DK Publishing, 2003.
Rippe, James N. *Heart Disease for Dummies.* Hoboken, N.J.: Wiley, 2004.

■ CIGARETTE ADDITIVES

Chemicals added to tobacco. The tobacco found in cigarettes is not pure. Tobacco companies take tobacco leaves and process them, adding several chemicals. These chemicals serve a variety of purposes, such as manipulating taste, strengthening the impact of **nicotine**, making the smoke more tolerable to the lungs, and masking secondhand smoke. Tobacco companies say additives are used to enhance flavor, make smoking more enjoyable, and separate their cigarettes from other brands. Doctors and opponents of the tobacco industry disagree. They argue that additives are used to increase the addictive nature of smoking, mask illnesses, and entice kids and teenagers into smoking.

THE SECRECY BEHIND CIGARETTE ADDITIVES

Tobacco companies keep their lists of additives secret. They argue that making these lists public would hurt their competitive edge over other companies. The tobacco companies are required to share their ingredients with the federal government. However, a confidentiality agreement does not allow the government to share this information with the public.

Most of our knowledge about cigarette additives comes from three sources. The first is a 1994 document provided by Brown and Williamson, once a large tobacco manufacturer in the United States (they merged with R.J. Reynolds in 2004). Brown and Williamson published a list of the 599 additives they used in their cigarettes. This is a master list of additives, meaning the company did not provide the specific combination of additives used for each cigarette brand they manufactured.

The second source of information comes from the British parliament. In 2000, the British parliament Select Committee on Health published a list of additives used in specific brands of cigarettes. The committee had requested the lists of additives used by five tobacco companies in Britain. Disregarding the companies' concerns about confidentiality, Parliament made these lists public. For the first time, consumers could know what additives are in the cigarettes they smoke. For example, additives in R.J. Reynolds's Camel Lights 84 mm include

- glycerol
- honey
- calcium carbonate
- cocoa
- propylene glycol
- guar gum
- licorice root, fluid, extract, and powder
- fruits, fresh, dried extracts, and esters thereof
- cellulose fiber
- flavorings
- maple syrup, extract, and concentrate
- polyvinyl alcohol
- citric acid and its tri-potassium and tri-sodium salts
- magnesium oxide

Although the additives in specific cigarette brands are listed, the amount of each additive used is still private.

The third source of information comes from the tobacco iudustry itself. In 1998, the four largest tobacco companies in the United States signed the Master Settlement Agreement (MSA) with 46 states and five U.S. territories. Part of the agreement involved making thousands of industry documents available to the public. This resulted in the creation of the Legacy Tobacco Documents Library. Reports, memos, letters, position statements, and other materials have been scanned and uploaded to the library. The public is able to view these documents for free at http://legacy.library.ucsf.edu. A great deal of tobacco-related research over the past decade has come from examining these documents.

REASONS ADDITIVES ARE USED

One reason companies use additives is to increase the amount of **freebase nicotine** found in cigarettes. Nicotine comes in two forms: bound and freebase. In its bound form, nicotine is attached to other smoke particles that enter the lungs. It takes longer for the body to absorb the nicotine from these particles. Freebase nicotine is not attached to other particles. When a cigarette is smoked, freebase nicotine is quickly absorbed by the lungs. The faster the nicotine is absorbed, the faster it reaches the brain. This means a smoker gets a stronger sensation (referred to as a kick or impact) from smoking a cigarette. Smokers want to continue to have this sensation—that's why they continue to smoke.

In a 1994 speech to the U.S. House Subcommittee on Health and Environment, Dr. David Kessler indicated that once nicotine enters the blood stream, it only takes seven to nine seconds to reach the brain, providing that "good" feeling. The nicotine interacts with chemicals in the brain, such as **dopamine**, that make people feel good. Because of this feeling, people want to re-create the experience. This leads to more smoking and a physical addiction to nicotine.

Q & A

Question: Are additives safe to use?

Answer: Individual additives are safe. The Brown and Williamson document listed 599 additives the company used in its cigarettes. The additives were classified as FEMA GRAS. This stands for "Generally Recognized As Safe by the Flavor and Extract Manufacturers Association." The controversy involves the reasons for using the additives and what happens when these chemicals are combined, lit, and smoked.

Critics of the tobacco industry argue that additives are used to dilate a smoker's airways. By dilating the airways, a smoker can take deeper breaths. More smoke is inhaled per puff. This means more nicotine can enter the lungs. If a cigarette has additives that open the airways and increase the amount of freebase nicotine, a smoker will receive a very strong kick. Tobacco companies disagree. They argue that the amount of additives found in cigarettes are not sufficient to dilate the airways.

Additives are also used to increase the social appeal of smoking. Even smokers agree that cigarette smoke is not pleasant. It irritates the eyes and lungs, causes clothing and hair to smell bad, and gives smokers bad breath. In a 2005 report in *Tobacco Control,* researchers discuss the attempt by tobacco companies to create more appealing cigarettes. This meant developing cigarettes that did not have a bad smell, cause bad breath, or give off side-stream smoke. Tobacco companies could not find the proper combination of additives to create socially acceptable cigarettes. In fact, many of the experiments produced cigarettes that even smokers did not want to touch.

Even though attempts to create the "socially acceptable" cigarettes did not work, the industry still experimented with additives to mask environmental tobacco smoke (ETS) (second-hand smoke, side-stream smoke). In a 2000 report in the journal *Tobacco Control,* researchers found that more than a dozen different additives were used to try and mask ETS.

EXAMPLES OF ADDITIVES

One way tobacco companies set themselves apart from others is the way their cigarettes taste. Without additives, cigarettes have a very harsh taste, and smokers cannot tolerate the smoke in their lungs. **Menthol** cigarettes are said to be "smooth" tasting. Menthol is a chemical that acts as a local anesthetic and can be found in peppermint, spearmint, and mint.

When added to tobacco, menthol provides a cooling sensation. Smokers will experience that sensation in their respiratory tracts. The irritation from the smoke will be less, and the cool sensation will feel good. Some critics of the tobacco industry say this helps mask the symptoms of respiratory diseases and ultimately causes more harm to a smoker.

In a 2006 study in *Nicotine and Tobacco Research,* researchers found that menthol cigarettes were the cigarettes of choice by both new and younger smokers. Critics argue that this contributes to the possibility of becoming addicted to smoking. The cooling sensation and taste will minimize the harshness of nicotine and reduce the urge to quit.

Additives can be added to the tobacco so that the smoke will contain more free-based nicotine. **Ammonia** is one additive known for doing this. Ammonia was first used by Philip Morris in its Marlboro brand of cigarettes. Ammonia alters the pH in smoke. The higher the pH level, the more smoke will contain freebase nicotine. The use of ammonia technology is credited for making Marlboro one of the top cigarette brands in the country. A 2004 paper in *Nicotine and Tobacco Research* highlights the controversies surrounding the use of ammonia. The tobacco industry argues that ammonia does not increase the addictiveness of nicotine. Researchers disagree, arguing that by increasing the freebase nicotine in cigarette smoke, people will enjoy the feeling more and be less likely to want to quit.

One additive that increases the addictive nature of nicotine is **acetaldehyde**. Acetaldehyde is created when sugar is burned. Add sugar to the tobacco mixture, and when a cigarette is lit, an acetaldehyde is formed. Scientists argue that nicotine and acetaldehyde work together to increase the addictiveness of nicotine. Tobacco companies state that sugar is used to help give cigarettes flavor.

Another additive tobacco companies use is **levulinic acid**. Nicotine smoke is harsh. To make smoking more enjoyable and reduce the harshness from smoking, this additive is mixed in with the tobacco. In a 2005 report in *Nicotine & Tobacco Research,* the authors found industry documents indicating tobacco companies know that levulinic acid acts as more than a flavor. A 1999 document by ASH (Action on Smoking and Health) also reviewed tobacco-industry documents. The organization argues that levulinic acid can be used to make the brain more receptive to nicotine. This increases the addictive power of smoking.

Fact Or Fiction?

The cocoa that is used in cigarettes can dilate a person's airways.

The Facts: Tobacco companies use cocoa as an additive because it gives cigarettes a stronger "kick." One of the chemicals found in cocoa is **theobromine**. Theobromine helps expand the airways in a person's lungs, allowing more nicotine to be rapidly absorbed. The tobacco industry claims there is not enough theobromine in a cigarette to expand the airways. Critics disagree. There is not enough scientific evidence to conclusively say which side is right.

CONTROVERSIES ABOUT USING ADDITIVES

The controversy surrounding additives is simple. Tobacco companies argue that additives are necessary for them to be able to sell a product that people will enjoy. They also have publicly stated that the additives they use do not harm consumers. Critics of the tobacco industry argue that additives are used to increase the addictiveness of smoking, hurt a smoker's body, and help mask, or hide, the damage caused by smoking.

Both sides have legitimate points. Additives are used to make tobacco products more appealing to consumers. However, documents found in the Legacy Tobacco Documents Library show that tobacco companies knew about the consequences of their additives.

Dr. Greg N. Connally of Harvard University testified before Congress about the use of additives in cigarettes. He stated:

> In 2002, RJR [R.J. Reynolds, a large producer of cigarettes] introduced Camel 'Exotic' Blends and Brown and Williamson 'Kool Fusion' brands all with candy-like flavors in the product. The Exalt Camel brand used a plastic pellet in the filter to deliver flavors to smokers. No public health agency knew it was present, its toxicity or how it contributed to youth initiation. Candy-like flavors mask the natural toxicity of smoke and could enhance initiation and addiction.

Of course, tobacco companies take issue with these types of statements. A memo by British American Tobacco that was submitted in 2000 to the Select Committee on Health in Britain's parliament stated:

> Ammonia compounds occur naturally in tobacco. Tobaccos contain natural ammonia compounds and sugars which react with one another during the curing and ageing processes . . . We add ammonia to some of our US-style cigarettes to enhance the reaction with sugars to further improve their flavour. Ammonia technology as such in commercial products does not increase 'smoke pH', does not boost nicotine delivery to smokers and does not otherwise increase the smokers' absorption of nicotine.

The Gallaher Group PLC also submitted a memo to Parliament, addressing their stance on the health risks of smoking. "Traditionally, additives have been used in the course of manufacture of tobacco products to improve product quality. Additives are essentially used by Gallaher both for technological purposes and to give individual products their distinctive flavour and aroma characteristics."

Tobacco industry documents reveal additives were used for more than just flavoring purposes. To help resolve the debate on the negative effects of cigarette additives, scientists will need to conduct more research.

See also: Addiction to Nicotine; The Body and Smoking; Withdrawal

FURTHER READING

Bates, Clive, Martin Jarvis, and Gregory Connolly. *Tobacco Additives: Cigarette Engineering and Nicotine Addiction.* Available online. URL: http://old.ash.org.uk/html/regulation/html/additives.html.

■ COSMETIC EFFECTS OF SMOKING

How the chemicals in smoke affect the appearance and detract from physical attractiveness. Smoking damages the skin, mouth, teeth, fingernails, and hair. Chemicals such as **nicotine, carbon monoxide,** formaldehyde, and arsenic, which are present in tobacco products, enter the bloodstream. They then work to alter one's physical appearance by, for example, adding wrinkles, discoloring skin complexion, and yellowing fingernails.

Secondhand smoke also causes cosmetic damage when it comes in contact with the body. The harm done to a person's appearance is gradual and may take years of smoking to create noticeable, lasting effects. Smokers who quit can prevent further damage to their physical features. However, in many cases, the years of damage inflicted on the skin cannot be repaired without cosmetic surgery.

SMOKING AND SKIN DAMAGE

Smoking hurts the skin in several ways. First, the lungs rapidly absorb chemicals and toxins from the smoke when it is inhaled. These chemicals then enter the bloodstream. The nicotine in smoke causes blood vessels to constrict, or narrow, throughout the body, This means the body, including the skin, does not receive enough oxygen, vitamins, and nutrients to function properly. Smoking just one cigarette can constrict blood vessels for up to 90 minutes. Smoking throughout the day causes **hypoxia,** a condition where the body is deprived of an adequate supply of oxygen.

Second, when blood vessels constrict, the blood that flows through them thickens. This reduces the amounts of collagen and elastin found in the skin. Collagen and elastin are proteins that help make up the skin and give it strength and durability. An adequate blood supply is needed to create and maintain healthy levels of collagen and elastin.

Third, smoke contains carbon monoxide, which is a poisonous gas. When inhaled, the carbon monoxide attaches itself to **hemoglobin,** a protein in red blood cells that carries oxygen. The carbon monoxide replaces most of the oxygen in hemoglobin. The hemoglobin then carries the toxic chemical throughout the body and further reduces the amount of oxygen the skin receives.

The internal and external damage from smoking results in several changes to a person's appearance. Smoking makes people look older than they are. The lack of collagen and elastin causes the skin to wrinkle, most notably on the face. Research published in the *Archives of Dermatology* in 2007, however, has shown that smoking promotes wrinkles all over the body, not only on the face. In a 2003 report, Britain's Chief Medical Officer stated that a smoker's skin can age by 10 to 20 years. Thus, a smoker who is 40 years old may appear to be 50 to 60 years old.

Q & A

Question: If I quit smoking, will the wrinkles in my skin disappear?

Answer: Once damaged, the wrinkles in the skin will not naturally disappear. Smokers who quit will help prevent further wrinkles from occurring. A person can undergo Botox treatments or cosmetic surgery to mask wrinkles or hopefully make them disappear. Over-the-counter products such as wrinkle- and anti-aging creams may provide some temporary help, depending on how wrinkled the face is.

Smoking causes skin wounds to heal more slowly. Blood, oxygen, collagen, and elastin work together to heal cuts and bruises. The internal and external damage caused by smoking means the body has to work harder and longer to repair injuries. Studies in the *Archives of*

Dermatology (1991), *Hand* (1977), and *Plastic Reconstructive Surgery* (1994), support this observation.

Fact Or Fiction?

Smoking won't damage my hair.

The Facts: In a 1996 study published in *British Medical Journal (BMJ)*, researchers found that smoking led both to hair prematurely turning gray and to hair loss. The chemicals in smoke are circulated throughout the whole body, including the scalp and hair follicles. The result is a premature graying of the hair. Also, in a 2007 study published in the *Archives of Dermatology,* the authors found that men who smoked at least 20 cigarettes a day had moderate or severe hair loss later in life.

Smokers can also develop the "nicotine sign." This refers to the yellow fingernails found on smokers. The nails most likely to be stained are the ones on the hand used to hold cigarettes. The chemical byproducts in the smoke stain the nails. When a person stops smoking the nicotine sign will eventually disappear. As fingernails continue to grow, the new part of the nails look normal. The stained part of the nails will shrink every time a person trims the fingernails.

Q & A

Question: What does the term *smoker's face* mean?

Answer: In 1985, a doctor in England coined the term *smoker's face* when he found he could identify smokers by looking at their faces. Some characteristics of smoker's face include lines or wrinkles, thin and bony facial features (such as hollow cheeks), yellow-gray skin color, and an older appearance.

SMOKING AND SKIN DISEASE

Smoking increases the risk of developing several skin diseases. Skin diseases often discolor parts of the skin and create lesions that can leave permanent scars.

Smoking and Psoriasis

Psoriasis is a chronic skin disease. The most common type is plaque psoriasis. This type of psoriasis causes raised, inflamed, red lesions with silvery scales on the skin. Once a person develops psoriasis, it becomes a life-long condition. The psoriasis can flare up and then go into remission. The other forms of psoriasis can affect larger areas of the skin, cause more serious inflammation, and have the potential to permanently scar the skin.

In a 2007 study published in the *American Journal of Medicine,* researchers found that women who smoked increased their risk of developing psoriasis by 78 percent, compared to nonsmoking women. Women who previously smoked, but quit, still had a 37 percent higher risk of getting psoriasis than women who did not smoke. The elevated risk of developing psoriasis returns to normal once a person stops smoking and stays smoke-free for 20 years.

The National Psoriasis Foundation reports that smoking also plays an important role in the remission of psoriasis. The foundation cites a study where 78 percent of people who experienced remissions were nonsmokers. By comparison, 22 percent of people who experienced remissions were smokers. When looking at people who never experienced a remission, 66 percent were smokers. The remaining 34 percent were nonsmokers.

Smoking and Squamous Cell Carcinoma

Smoking has been linked to numerous cancers, including skin cancer. There are several types of skin cancer: squamous cell carcinoma, melanoma, and basal cell carcinoma. Although there is an established link between smoking and a variety of cancers, research is still being conducted on the relationships between smoking and skin cancers. However, a clear connection has been found between smoking and squamous cell carcinoma. In a 2001 study published in the *Journal of Clinical Oncology,* the authors showed that current smokers are three times as likely to develop squamous cell carcinoma as nonsmokers. Former smokers are almost twice as likely to develop squamous cell carcinoma than nonsmokers.

Squamous cell carcinoma occurs when cancer cells invade the upper layer of the skin. Lesions can develop and damage the skin. Squamous cell carcinoma is very treatable when detected early. It is harder to treat if early detection is missed because there is a greater potential for it to have spread to a much larger area.

SMOKING AND ORAL HEALTH

The same processes that harm the skin also harm the mouth. Restricted blood flow and exposure to smoke damage the teeth, lips, tongue, and cheeks. First, smoking stains the teeth. The stains can range from yellow to dark brown to gray. The nicotine and other chemicals in the smoke stick to the teeth. Over time, the chemicals erode the white enamel and turn it yellow. The color will continue to darken as long as a person continues to smoke.

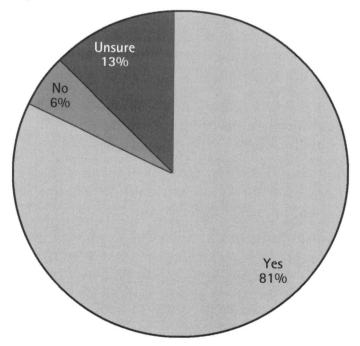

DID YOU KNOW?

Survey of Periodontists

Do people who smoke have less attractive smiles than people who don't smoke?

Unsure 13%

No 6%

Yes 81%

In a 2000 survey, periodontists were asked if they felt smoking hurt their patients' smiles. The great majority felt people who smoked had less attractive smiles.

Source: American Academy of Periodontology Online Survey of Periodontists, 2000.

Smokers are more likely than nonsmokers to develop tooth decay, chronic gum disease, and lose teeth. Oral wounds also take longer to heal in smokers. Gum diseases such as **gingivitis** and **periodontitis** are often painless and go unnoticed until a dental exam. In a 2000 study in the *Journal of Periodontology,* researchers found that among current smokers, 74.8 percent of periodontitis was caused by smoking. They estimated that 41.9 percent of all periodontitis cases in the United States can be attributed to current smoking behavior. Another 10.9 percent of all cases can be attributed to prior smoking. This means that more than 50 percent of all periodontitis cases are a result of smoking.

The toxins that enter the blood stream also destroy the bones that hold teeth in place. Thus, the combination of gum disease and weakened bones contributes to tooth loss. In a 2007 study in Japan, researchers found that current smokers were almost twice as likely to lose at least one tooth as nonsmokers.

Smokers, particularly male smokers, can develop a black hairy tongue. The top of the tongue has a furry brown-black look to it, Although the tongue looks horrible, it is not painful. Gently brushing the tongue can help the tongue return to normal. Dentists may also prescribe certain types of mouthwash or antibiotics to help cure the condition.

Oral cancer is another risk associated with smoking. The cancer can create painful lesions in the mouth. The cancer can disfigure the lips and tongue and contribute to tooth loss. If a cancerous lesion is on the inside of the cheek, the lesion may eat through the tissue to the skin, disfiguring the cheek. The American Cancer Society reports that 90 percent of people with oral cancer use some form of tobacco. The Cleveland Clinic states that smokers are six times more likely than nonsmokers to develop oral cancer.

More than 30 years of research has established the fact that smoking can harm one's appearance. The chemicals in smoke reduce the body's ability to maintain the blood flow necessary to nourish the skin and mouth. Exposure to secondhand smoke stains the teeth and fingernails, while making the skin brittle. Doctors report the best action for smokers to take is to stop smoking. Nonsmokers should not start smoking and do their best to avoid secondhand smoke.

See also: The Body and Smoking; The Mouth and Smoking.

FURTHER READING

May, Suellen. *Botox and Other Cosmetic Drugs.* New York: Chelsea House, 2008.

■ COST OF SMOKING

Financial impact of smoking. The cost of smoking goes beyond paying for tobacco products. A smoker can count on having higher medical bills, lost wages, higher insurance costs, and spending more on cosmetics and clothing. Smoking-related illnesses cost tens of billions every year. These costs are paid for by individuals, insurance companies, and both the state and federal governments. Government-related costs are ultimately paid by the taxpayers.

COST TO SMOKE

Smoking is a big business in the United States. The Centers for Disease Control and Prevention (CDC) report that $82 billion was spent on cigarette purchases in 2005. A total of $88.8 billion was spent in 2005 for all tobacco purchases. In a 2005 report in *Consumer Expenditure Survey Anthology,* researchers estimate that the average U.S. smoker spends $1,321 each year on tobacco products. Heavy smokers pay much more than that. As the price of cigarettes continues to rise, smokers will spend even more money to continue their habit.

According to the Campaign for Tobacco-Free Kids, the average retail price for a pack of cigarettes is $4.63. Smokers in New Jersey pay the most, at $6.51 per pack. Smokers in South Carolina pay only $3.41 per pack, which is lower than anywhere else in the country. Approximately half of the cost is due to federal cigarette taxes, state cigarette taxes, and state sales tax.

Research has shown that every time the price of cigarettes rises, the number of smokers drops. The reason is that many smokers cannot afford to continue the habit. They are forced to quit. However, many smokers seek out alternatives to quitting. In a 2005 study in *Tobacco Control,* researchers found that smokers often look for places where cigarettes are less expensive. This includes going to Native American reservations or other states and counties where the taxes on cigarettes are lower. Another option is to smoke generic or lower quality cigarettes.

Fact Or Fiction?

People who can least afford to smoke are the ones who smoke the most.

The Facts: Research has repeatedly shown that people in the lower socioeconomic classes smoke more than people in the upper socioeconomic classes. Relatively speaking, it costs people with less income more to smoke than wealthier people. People in lower income brackets are also less likely to have health insurance. This means they must pay in full for their

DID YOU KNOW?

Annual Smoking-Attributable Economic Costs for Adults and Infants—United States, 1995–1999

Cost component	Total (in millions)	Per smoker*
Adult costs		
Annual smoking-attributable productivity costs, 1995–1999		
Men	$55,389	$2,278
Women	$26,483	$1,193
Total	$81,872	$1,760
Smoking-attributable medical expenditures, 1998**		
Ambulatory care	$27,182	$584
Hospital care	$17,140	$368
Prescription drugs	$6,364	$137
Nursing home	$19,383	$417
Other care	$5,419	$116
Total	$75,488	$1,623
Total adult costs	$157,360	$3,383
Infant costs		
Smoking-attributable neonatal medical expenditures, 1996	$366	$704
Total costs	$157,726	$3,391

* Approximately 46.5 million U.S. residents aged > 18 years smoked in 1999 (24,316,033 men and 22,199,233 women), based on the civilian noninstitutional population and respondents from the 1999 National Health Interview Survey. Smoking-attributable neonatal expenditures are per maternal smoker; average costs per adult smoker were approximately $8. Total productivity costs are weighted averages for men and women. Totals may not equal sum because of rounding.

**Data sources: Expenditure smoking-attributable fractions cited in reference 8 and 1998 personal health-care expenditure data obtained from the Centers for Medicare and Medicaid Services. Annual smoking-related medical costs were $157 billion, with each smoker being responsible for $3,391.

Source: Centers for Disease Control and Prevention.

medical bills. These smokers, therefore, are hurt twice by smoking: once for buying the cigarettes and again for the health problems cigarettes cause.

MEDICAL COSTS

Billions of dollars are spent every year on smoking-related illnesses. The Centers for Disease Control and Prevention (CDC) estimates that smoking is responsible for at least $165 billion in disability and health-care costs each year. Thus, individuals, insurance companies, and both state and local governments spend that amount every year to cover costs that are preventable.

In a 2003 CDC report, researchers found the most common smoking-attributable conditions for current and former smokers are: chronic bronchitis, emphysema, heart attacks, all cancers *except* lung, strokes, and then lung cancer. In another CDC report, published in 2005, researchers found that the following were the top three smoking-attributable diseases that led to death from 1997 to 2001: lung cancer, **chronic obstructive pulmonary disease**, and **ischemic heart disease**.

These smoking-related diseases cost insurance companies a huge amount of money. In a 2007 study in the *American Journal of Health Behavior,* the authors examined insurance claims from large employers for the years 1996 through 2001. They found the greatest number of insurance claims occurred for ischemic heart disease. Expenses for inpatient, outpatient, and prescriptions cost $263 million during the first year following a diagnosis of ischemic heart disease. Another $152 million was spent to cover the same services during the second year of treatment. Insurance companies paid out approximately $176 million over two years for expenditures related to chronic obstructive pulmonary disease. For lung cancer patients, insurance companies paid $62 million for health-care expenses. This leads insurance companies to increase the price of health insurance policies. Then workers and their employers have to pay more for health insurance.

Examining health-care costs at the state level provides another picture of the impact smoking has on society. In a 2004 study in *Tobacco Control,* the authors report that the total costs of smoking in California in 1999 came to $15.9 billion. Medical costs accounted for $8.6 billion to cover hospital care, ambulatory care, home health care, nursing home care, and prescriptions. Missouri, a much smaller state than California, spent $1.67 billion in 1998 on health-care costs.

Taxpayers also have to shoulder the costs related to smoking. A 2005 fact sheet distributed by the Campaign for Tobacco-Free Kids reports that U.S. households pay an average of $456 per year to help the federal government pay for smoking-caused expenses. That comes out to $49.5 billion every year. These include smoking-related health-care costs covered by Medicare, Medicaid, and the Veterans Affairs health-care system. Thus, the general public pays a steep price to provide health care for smoking-related illnesses.

Pediatric medical costs

Secondhand smoke contributes to health-care costs, especially for children who are more susceptible to smoking-related illnesses. In a 2007 report from the University of Maine, researchers examined the economic impact of secondhand smoke on children. They estimate that approximately $8 million to $11.5 million per year is spent on health-care costs for child illnesses related to secondhand smoke exposure. It is estimated that $2.4 million is for childhood asthma. Another $2 million a year is spent treating pneumonia, and $1.5 million to treat wheezing.

In a 2007 study in the *Journal of Health Care Finance,* researchers estimate that $640 million to $860 million in pediatric health-care costs can be attributed to smoking in the household. Expenses for respiratory illnesses were higher in households with smokers. The same was true for hospital-related expenses.

In a 2002 study in *Health Economics,* researchers examined **neonatal** health-care costs as a result of women who smoked during pregnancy. Babies born to women who smoked were approximately 20 percent more likely to be admitted to a neonatal intensive care unit (NICU) and stayed longer than babies born to nonsmoking mothers. The nightly cost to be in a NICU is almost $2,500, compared to $748 for infants in a nursery. The cost to the United States was approximately $367 million in 1996 (adjusted for inflation, that comes to $495 million in 2007 dollars).

COSTS TO EMPLOYERS

Companies spend a great deal of money to insure employees. In a 2007 report by the Kaiser Family Foundation, researchers found the average annual cost of health insurance for an employee wanting single coverage (no child/family coverage) was $4,497. This number jumps to $12,106 every year to provide family coverage. Employers pay the bulk of the premiums. The researchers found that companies paid 84 percent of the premium for employees with single coverage and paid 72 percent of the premium for employees with family coverage.

Q & A

Why can insurance companies charge companies whose employees smoke higher premiums?

Answer: Premiums are based, in part, on how much money individuals cost insurance companies. The more medical bills a person has, the more an insurance company has to pay to health-care providers. Like any business that relies on profits, insurance companies are in the business of making money. Therefore, they charge people higher premiums for having more medical expenses. As a result, companies with more smokers pay more to offer this benefit to their employees.

Companies, especially small and midsize companies, are essentially penalized for having employees who smoke. The CDC estimates that smokers have $1,623 in excess medical expenses, which in turn cost employers more money because of increased insurance premiums. The North Carolina Department of Health and Human Services reports that each employee who smokes costs an employer $1,429 per year in additional health-care costs.

Q & A

Question: Are there other ways employees who smoke cause companies to lose money?

Answer: Smokers are less productive at work than nonsmokers. They also are absent twice as much as nonsmokers. The Centers for Disease Control and Prevention (CDC) estimates that productivity losses due to smoking- and secondhand smoke–related deaths are $92 billion per year. In a 2004 study in *Tobacco Control*, researchers found that smoking related illnesses accounted for $1.5 billion in lost productivity. This does not even take into account how much employers lose because of reduced productivity and employee absenteeism.

OTHER COSTS

There are other expenses that smokers have to assume that have no set dollar amount. Smoking damages many things, including the smoker's skin and teeth and clothing, furniture, and other personal belongings. Over-the-counter cosmetic treatments and cosmetic surgery can be expensive. The costs of replacing clothing and furniture can add up. Fires started by cigarettes can displace people from their homes and cause thousands of dollars in damage.

Smokers pay more in life insurance costs. The North Carolina Department of Health and Human Services reports that one insurance company offers a $500,000 life insurance policy to 30-year-old nonsmokers for $425 year. The same policy for smokers is $935. In addition, homeowners or renters insurance is often higher for smokers. An estimated 23,000 residential fires occur every year. Smokers can count on having even higher insurance premiums if they file a claim that is related to smoking.

The National Fire Protection Agency reports that in 2005 there were approximately 82,400 fires started by smoking materials (lighted cigarettes, cigars, pipes, and so forth). This resulted in 800 deaths, 1,660 injuries, and $575 million in property damage. Twenty-five percent of those who died were not the smokers whose cigarettes started the fires.

Smoking-related diseases kill people. Economists create estimates to how much money is lost because of both smoking-related illnesses and smoking-related deaths. In a 2005 report by the CDC, researchers examined the years of potential life lost and productivity losses due to smoking for the years between 1997 and 2001. They found that exposure to tobacco smoke accounted for approximately 438,000 deaths per year. Each year, these deaths account for 5.5 million years of potential life lost. This figure reflects the total number of years these victims would have lived.

FURTHER READING
Sloan, Frank A. *The Price of Smoking.* Boston: MIT Press, 2004.

■ DRUGS AND TOBACCO USE

The U.S. government has banned highly addictive drugs that affect mood, concentration, and/or behavior. Illicit drugs include marijuana, amphetamines (speed), cocaine, and heroin. Research into drug dependency shows that for some teenagers, cigarette smoking is often the first step toward the use of illegal drugs.

The government has used several methods to assess how many young people are involved with drugs. One effort has been "Monitoring the Future," an annual study sponsored by the National Institute on Drug Abuse (NIDA). NIDA polls more than 40,000 students each year for information on drug use and attitudes toward drugs. According to figures for 2007, 35.9 percent of students in the 12th grade had used an illicit drug in the previous year. More than 31 percent had used marijuana in the previous year, and more than 66 percent had used alcohol. According to the survey, 21.6 percent of the 12th graders had smoked cigarettes during the previous month, and more than 44 percent also had used alcohol.

NICOTINE: A GATEWAY DRUG

For young people, alcohol and **nicotine** are two of the most easily obtained drugs. Beer and cigarettes can be found in many homes. Along with marijuana and inhalants, alcohol and nicotine are considered **gateway drugs**, substances that introduce people to drug abuse and can lead to the use of more serious drugs.

Fact Or Fiction?

It's just a cigarette—smoking isn't about doing drugs.

The Facts: For a majority of smokers, this statement may be true. But consider that almost 45 percent of teenagers who use drugs other than marijuana also smoke. For a troubling number of people, cigarette smoking is often the first indicator of a willingness to take risks with their health.

For many years, cigarette smoking has been used to predict the likelihood of people using other drugs. In a 2007 report by Columbia University's Center on Addiction and Substance Abuse (CASA), researchers revealed some startling information on teenage smoking and drug use. The study focused on teenagers who were 12 to 17 years old. The researchers found that teenage smokers are more than

8.5 times more likely to currently use illicit drugs than nonsmoking teens. It turns out that more than 63 percent of teenage marijuana smokers also smoke cigarettes. For teenagers who actively use drugs other than marijuana, almost 45 percent also smoke cigarettes. Additionally, 92 percent of active teenage heroin users also smoke cigarettes. Although fewer than 1 percent of teenagers smoke heroin, almost all who do also smoke cigarettes.

A 2008 report by the Substance Abuse and Mental Health Services (part of the U.S. Department of Health and Human Services) found that people addicted to nicotine were more likely to use other drugs than those without the addiction. According to the data, 40.1 percent of those with nicotine addictions engaged in binge drinking compared to 20.1 percent of those without this addiction. Only 5.5 percent of people without a nicotine addiction engaged in heavy drinking, compared to 14.9 percent of people with an addiction. Illicit drug use was also more common among those with a nicotine addiction—20.7 percent compared to 6.2 percent.

The American Academy of Pediatrics (AAP), a national organization of medical professionals who treat young people, issued a warning to parents on the subject of gateway drugs: "While using alcohol and tobacco, young people develop behaviors that can also be associated with using drugs, such as a willingness to take chances."

According to the AAP, using tobacco and alcohol teaches young people:

- how to obtain substances illegally;
- how much of the substance to use;
- how to control the side effects;
- how to hide what they've done and lie about it; and
- how to deal with any guilt and shame over what they've done.

The AAP is not saying that use of tobacco and alcohol causes young people to use harder drugs. The AAP is saying that the use of alcohol and tobacco "sets up patterns of behavior that may make it easier to take the next step and use other drugs."

Simply mastering the art of smoking is an important stepping-stone to other drugs. Smoking is, after all, an unnatural act—inhaling a substance that makes one choke. A 1972 Canadian government report on drugs noted that inhaling smoke is difficult and unpleasant for the starting smoker. He or she needs considerable practice to control the reflex to choke or cough. Before a person can take pleasure from smoking, this natural obstacle must be overcome. Then, as the report puts it, "the general 'smoking barrier' is removed, and the smoker is then more likely to try smoking other drugs."

PLAYING WITH FIRE

Young people tend to live in the moment, without much thought for the future. As they reach their teenage years, they discover a wider world, with many new opportunities—and dangers. Sometimes you may hear about teens who "experiment" with drugs and alcohol, as if they were in a chemistry lab. Unfortunately, their laboratories are their own bodies. Still worse, these young people move on to perform more risky experiments.

Since 1991, the Centers for Disease Control and Prevention (CDC) has monitored the chances young people take with their health through the Youth Risk Behavior Surveillance System (YRBSS). It is a nationwide survey of selected students from the seventh through the 12th grades. Students answer a variety of questions on subjects that concern their health and well-being, including, tobacco use, unhealthy lifestyles, alcohol and drug use, sexual behavior, and activities that lead to injury or violence.

Studies also show smokers are more likely than nonsmokers to use alcohol and illicit drugs. According to a 2007 issue of *Psychiatrische Praxis,* a European study found that smokers in the ninth grade also are more likely to drink. In fact, compared to nonsmokers, smokers are three times more likely to drink alcohol and four times more likely to binge drink. Smokers were also more likely to have used marijuana—40 percent compared to 6 percent among nonsmokers.

The authors of a 2005 study published in *Biological Pyschiatry* looked at smoking as a gateway drug for those with and without attention deficit hyperactivity disorder (ADHD). Twenty-two percent of youth with ADHD were smokers, compared to 12 percent of those without ADHD. For both groups, smoking was found to be a gateway drugs. Youth who smoked were more likely to use other drugs, including alcohol, marijuana, and other drugs (cocaine, amphetamines, sedatives, and so forth). However, these findings were stronger for those with ADHD. This means that smokers with

ADHD were more likely than smokers without ADHD to try alcohol and drugs.

According to adolescent smoking statistics issued by the Substance Abuse and Mental Health Services Administration in 2007, 3.1 million young people smoke in the United States. With so many youthful smokers potentially at risk, one can understand the emphasis former surgeon general Joycelyn Elders put on smoking, "This is one of the few early warning signs we have in public health. If we can prevent tobacco use in the first place, we might have a big impact on preventing or delaying a host of other destructive behaviors among our young people."

Q & A

Question: I've got a friend who's trying to quit smoking, but it's driving him crazy. Lately, he's been saying, "I can smoke just one." Is he right?

Answer: Your friend is right if he wants to cut down on his smoking but not if he wants to stop. The web site for the University of Maryland Medical Center, which discusses the problems in quitting, notes that people who cheat in the first two weeks of quitting almost always ended up smoking again. Nearly one-half of those who successfully resisted cheating were still smoke-free in six months.

If your friend gives in on "just one," he'll soon end up smoking his regular dose. See if you can help him find some other distraction. Maybe you can check if there's any counseling available to help him keep on the smoke-free road.

See also: Alcohol and Tobacco Use; Medications and Smoking

FURTHER READING
Bellenir, Karen, ed. *Substance Abuse Sourcebook.* Detroit: Omnigraphics, 1996.
Lowinson, Joyce H., Pedro Ruiz, Robert B. Millman, and John G. Langrod. *Substance Abuse: A Comprehensive Textbook, 4th Edition.* New York: Lippincott Williams & Wilkins, 2004.
Miller, William R., and Kathleen M. Carroll. *Rethinking Substance Abuse: What the Science Shows, and What We Should Do About It.* New York: Guilford Press, 2007.

■ GOVERNMENT AND TOBACCO

At all levels of government, tobacco use creates complex problems. Tobacco companies are large businesses that provide jobs and pay taxes that support many government programs. However, they also produce a product that has endangered millions of people over the years, burdening society with enormous costs for not only lost wages and productivity but also health care.

TOBACCO AND THE FEDERAL GOVERNMENT

At the national level, the government has helped the tobacco business. Major tobacco companies have also influenced federal laws and regulatory policy.

International trade

According to the U.S. Constitution, the federal government has the power to regulate not only trade among the states but also trade with other nations. Tobacco has long played an important role in international trade. It was the first major American export crop. It remains an important crop. In the 1980s, for example, facing a decline in sales at home, American companies tried to boost exports of cigarettes. When they encountered barriers in foreign markets, they approached the trade officials in the federal government for help. Their proposals found a receptive audience. For many years, the United States has purchased more goods from foreign countries than it sells. Trade officials were eager to find products that would help to reduce those losses. Government officials pressured Japan, Thailand, and South Korea to open their markets or lower import taxes to improve sales of American cigarettes. As a result, American companies were exporting 243 billion cigarettes by 1996. By 2006, the number of cigarettes had dropped to 109.9 billion at a value of $1.2 billion.

In recent years, the World Health Organization (WHO), the international public health agency of the United Nations, has become concerned over the rising sales of cigarettes around the world. To deal with the connected rise in health problems, WHO proposed a treaty for worldwide control of tobacco sales and advertising. By June 2008, 168 nations had signed, including the United States.

Tobacco subsidies

A **subsidy** is a grant made by the government to an enterprise that benefits the public. To help the nation's farmers, the federal government manages a complicated system of subsidies that control how much they can sell and at what price. Those subsidies include tobacco farmers. The Environmental Working Group found that the government spent $530 million on tobacco subsidies from 2000 through 2004. Federal legislation eliminated these subsidies at the end of the 2004 tobacco crop year. Therefore, tax money is no longer being spent to support tobacco farming.

Antismoking activists, however, point out that even more money is spent on indirect subsidies. Smokers suffer from cancer, heart attacks, strokes, and lung diseases. The government pays for much of their medical care. Medicare is a system of health-care insurance for the elderly and permanently disabled, funded by the federal government. Medicaid is the health-care program that assists people with low incomes and is paid for by both federal and state governments. According to the Centers for Medicare and Medicaid Services, the federal government spent $408.3 billion on Medicare in 2006. Another $210.1 billion was spent on Medicaid programs. Those percentages may sound small, but Medicare costs the federal government $432 billion a year and its share of Medicaid costs came to $181.7 billion. The federal government also pays additional expenses for smoking-related health care through organizations like the Veterans Administration and the Department of Defense.

STATE GOVERNMENTS AND TOBACCO

States also bear at least some of the costs of tobacco-related illnesses. As previously stated, each state is also responsible for Medicaid costs. According to the Organization for Tobacco-Free Kids, the 2006 bill for tobacco-related Medicaid costs for all 50 states was more than $13.3 billion, with additional state costs of $2.9 billion. Total tobacco-related health costs were more than $70 billion.

In 1995, Mississippi attorney general Michael Moore decided to sue the large tobacco companies to recover his state's costs for treating people with tobacco-related illnesses. The other 49 states filed their own suits. Over the course of several years, the states and Big Tobacco negotiated, finally coming to an out-of-court settlement in November 1998.

The tobacco companies agreed to pay 46 of the states included in the settlement more than $200 billion over 25 years. In addition, the companies accepted new restrictions on advertising and sales of cigarettes to young people. Special payments were arranged for tobacco farmers. Tobacco companies even agreed to fund a new organization, the American Legacy Foundation, to educate people about the dangers of smoking. The tobacco companies resolved the lawsuits of four other states, Mississippi, Florida, Texas, and Minnesota, separately.

The Master Settlement Agreement, as the settlement with the 46 states came to be called, was the largest legal settlement in history. The amount of money to be paid under the agreement staggered many people. As the settlement was announced, a variety of innovative new antismoking programs were proposed. It seemed as if a whole new era was beginning.

Some states established trust funds, investing their settlement payments so that earnings would continue to provide money for various antismoking programs even after the payments themselves stop. But by 2002, more than one-half of the settlement payments were being diverted to purposes other than health care.

As hard economic times hit the country, tax revenues fell, but the expenses of running government programs remained the same. States began to look at tobacco settlement money as a way to fill in budget gaps. Wisconsin, facing the worst fiscal situation in the state's history, sold off its $5.9 billion settlement for a one-time payment of $1.3 billion—enough to balance the budget for one year.

The tobacco settlement payments are arranged much the way lottery payments are. The money is usually paid off over a long time span, 20 or 25 years. However, the recipient can take a single lump-sum payment—but it will be much less. For states, this financial arrangement is called securitization. States offer bonds (securities) to raise funds now, which will be paid off with settlement money received in future years.

While Wisconsin is so far the only state to mortgage its whole settlement, other states, like Washington and New Jersey, have sold a portion of their funds. Cash-strapped California securitized 10 years of payments to raise $4.5 billion.

WHERE SHOULD THE MONEY GO?

Some organizations believed the money from the Master Settlement Agreement should be used only to pay for health care for tobacco-related illnesses. Other groups, notably the American Cancer Society, argued that the settlement money should also pay for tobacco control programs to reduce smoking.

Many states have devoted a portion of the money for antismoking programs. Hawaii and Texas are setting aside a percentage of their yearly settlement payments for trust funds with income from the investment devoted to antismoking programs. Connecticut invested several years of payments into a trust fund, with the proceeds going not only to smoking reduction programs but also toward a freeze in tuition costs for its state university. Alabama will use its payments to fund a $50 million program to bring manufacturing facilities to the state.

Several southern states have decided to devote portions of their settlement money to help tobacco farmers. North Carolina chose to put one-half of its $4.6 billion tobacco settlement into a trust fund. The profits are then given as grants to poor rural counties in the state. Tobacco farmers are also eligible for grants. Tobacco has long been the state's leading cash crop. Hard economic times and a steep drop in tobacco prices and growing quotas have hit the state's farmers hard.

North Carolina set up Golden LEAF (Long-term Economic Advancement Foundation) in 1999 as a nonprofit corporation. Golden LEAF has tried to help tobacco farmers diversify their crops. With grants from Golden LEAF, some tobacco farmers have experimented with growing grapes, and North Carolina's wineries are beginning to win awards. Other choices include hot peppers for use in organic insecticides, herbs for the natural health market, and exotic mushrooms. Farmers are also experimenting with raising goats and pasture-fed hogs.

The foundation is also supporting new farm products. Grants have helped pay for a blast-freezer for blueberries, an egg-processing plant, research in uses for sweet potatoes, and marketing help for wheat crops and selling goat meat. A local college received funding to set up an agribusiness center in its business school that will not only expand educational opportunities but also serve as an information resource for farmers statewide.

Among the millions of dollars distributed by Golden LEAF are a number of educational grants, including one to improve Internet access for rural counties and another to train and keep teachers in rural areas. The fund has also offered college scholarships to students from the poorest and most tobacco-dependent counties.

Q & A

Question: The government keeps putting more taxes on cigarettes, and the price of a pack just keeps rising. How do I quit?

Answer: Learn all you can about nicotine, how it affects you, and how you'll feel when you quit. You'll have a better chance of succeeding if you know what you're facing.

Use a quit journal to vent your feelings, especially when withdrawal makes you grouchy. You may want to start off with a list of reasons for stopping, to remind yourself when you're tempted to smoke.

Finally, see your doctor, and tell him or her what you're planning. You may get some good help, advice, or warnings before you make your attempt. Good luck!

POLITICIANS AND TOBACCO

Like other businesses, tobacco companies influence elected officials, especially federal and state lawmakers. They also hire **lobbyists**, professional representatives to influence policy and laws in the industry's best interest.

If they want to be elected—or stay in office—politicians need votes and money to campaign for votes. At a time when TV ads are often necessary to clinch even local elections, the cost of campaigning is very high.

Estimates vary on the number of workers directly involved with the tobacco industry. In 1994, the Tobacco Industry Research Committee stated that the tobacco industry was responsible for almost 2 million jobs. The TIRC was funded by tobacco companies and disbanded in 1998 as part of the Master Settlement Agreement. A 2000 report by the USDA Economic Research Service estimated that between 1.8 million and 3.1 million jobs were directly related to tobacco. Another 1 million to 2 million jobs were indirectly related to tobacco.

Tobacco companies are also major taxpayers. Estimates of federal tax on cigarettes for 2006 came to $7.3 billion. States and localities received an estimated $14 billion in cigarette tax revenue for 2007.

The Center for Responsive Politics, a government watchdog group, compiled statistics on political giving. Under federal election law, corporations are forbidden to make contributions out of their own treasuries, but they can contribute to political action committees

(PACs). In addition, executives and employees can make private donations. Between 1979 and 1990, an 11-year-period, tobacco companies contributed $1 million to political action committees for elections to federal offices. In 1995, the tobacco industry began to face the lawsuits that would lead to the Master Settlement Agreement, as well as attempts in Congress to impose new regulations on the business. In the five years between 1995 and the 2000 presidential race, tobacco PAC contributions shot up to $6.2 million. That represents more than double the previous rate of giving. The Center for Responsible Politics found that total tobacco-related political contributions between 1995 and 2000 came to $23.2 million. Action on Smoking and Health (ASH), an antismoking group, reported that $32 million had gone from tobacco companies to candidates and parties between 1995 and 2000.

Until 2002, "hard money" given to candidates faced federal regulation, but "soft money" given to political parties did not. A new campaign finance law limiting "soft money" came into effect in 2003, and tobacco companies gave only $1.1 million in contributions in the first nine months of that year.

According to a joint report by Common Cause and the Tobacco-Free Kids Action Fund, tobacco companies distributed more than $3.8 million in political contributions during the 2005–2006 election cycle. The tobacco industry spends even more money on **lobbying**. In 2006, the industry spent $18 million on professional lobbying firms and inhouse lobbyists.

A BALANCE OF POWER

Governments have been forced to balance support for the tobacco industry against the costs involved with treatment of tobacco-related illnesses. Governments have also considered the costs, both political and monetary, of tobacco regulation vs. the benefits of tax revenues generated by tobacco.

Tobacco companies have shrewdly used their resources to influence government policies at the federal and state levels. The threat of action through the judicial branch—the nation's court system—presented tobacco companies with a major setback in the form of the Master Settlement Agreement. Yet with the help of lobbyists, the tobacco companies have maintained allies in the executive and legislative branches and influence in all levels of government.

See also: Smoking and Society; Tobacco Worldwide

FURTHER READING

Brizer, David. *Quitting Smoking for Dummies.* New York: Wiley, 2003.

Dirthick, Martha A. *Up In Smoke: From Legislation to Litigation in Tobacco Politics.* Washington, D.C.: CQ Press, 2004.

Warner, Kenneth E., Stephen L. Isaacs, and James R. Knickman. *Tobacco Control Policy.* Hoboken, N.J.: Jossey-Bass, 2006.

■ HEALTH INSURANCE AND SMOKING

How smoking impacts health insurance options. Health insurance is a necessity in today's society. Medical expenses continue to rise, and people need health insurance to help pay for these costs. Because smokers are at higher risk for various illnesses and diseases, smokers are more likely than nonsmokers to have medical bills. Insurance companies pass on these expenses by charging higher premiums. Businesses, and small businesses in particular, that offer health insurance are penalized for having workers who smoke. As a result, many businesses now refuse to hire smokers, require employees who smoke to go through cessation—or quitting—programs, or require smokers pay for a greater percentage of their health insurance.

THE NEED FOR HEALTH INSURANCE

Health care is expensive. The National Coalition on Health Care estimates that $2.3 trillion was spent on health care in 2007. According to the Agency for Health Care Research and Quality, 84.7 percent of the U.S. population had some health-care expenses in 2004. For those who needed medical service, the average amount spent in 2004 was $3,879.

In a 2008 report by Milliman, Inc., researchers found that American families with four members had $14,500 worth of medical costs in 2007. Families without health insurance are responsible for the entire bill, while families with insurance only pay for a portion of it.

DID YOU KNOW?

Mean Annual Expense Per Person, by Type of Service, 2004

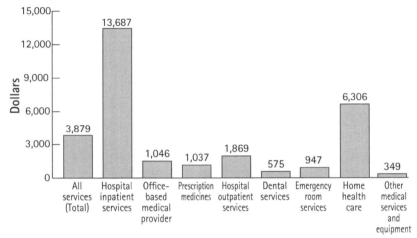

The average cost for different types of medical expenses varies greatly. Inpatient hospital services have the highest average, while "other medical services and equipment" has the lowest average.

Source: Center for Financing, Access, and Cost Trends, AHRQ, Household Component of the Medical Expenditure Panel Survey, 2004

Insurance is designed to protect people from the financial consequences of illnesses and accidents. For example, car insurance will help cover your car repair and medical costs if you are in a car accident. Health insurance works the same way. When you become ill or injured, the insurance company is there to protect you from what may be devastatingly high medical bills.

In order to receive this financial protection, people must pay insurance companies a yearly premium. Premiums are based on risk. People who are not likely to use their insurance will have lower premiums. If an insurance company believes a person is likely to use his or her coverage, the person will have to pay a higher premium. Insurance companies can deny coverage to people they feel are too great a risk.

MEDICAL COSTS

Billions of dollars are spent every year on smoking-related illnesses. The Centers for Disease Control and Prevention (CDC) estimates that smoking is responsible for at least $165 billion in disability and health-care costs every year.

In a 2005 CDC report, researchers found that the top three smoking-related diseases that led to death from 1997 through 2001 were: lung cancer, **chronic obstructive pulmonary disease,** and **ischemic heart disease.** These smoking-related diseases cost insurance companies millions of dollars every year.

In a 2007 study in the *American Journal of Health Behavior,* researchers found the greatest number of insurance claims were for ischemic heart disease. The study examined insurance data from large employers between 1996 and 2001. Expenses for inpatient care, outpatient care, and prescriptions cost health insurance companies $263 million during the first year following a diagnosis of ischemic heart disease. Another $152 million was spent by health insurance companies to cover the same services during the second year of treatment. Insurance companies also paid out approximately $176 million over two years for expenses related to chronic obstructive pulmonary disease. For lung cancer patients, insurance companies paid $62 million for health-care expenses over two years.

In a 2007 study in the *Journal of Preventative Medicine and Public Health,* the authors examined smoking-related medical expenses in Korea. In 2003, $74.2 million was spent treating lung cancer. The cost of treating smoking-related strokes was $65.3 million, while $50.1 million was spent treating chronic obstructive pulmonary disease (COPD).

OBTAINING HEALTH INSURANCE

In general, there are three ways a person can obtain health insurance: purchase it directly, obtain it through an employer, or sign up for a government health plan such as Medicaid. Purchasing health insurance is very expensive. An insurance company will evaluate your overall health, any preexisting conditions you may have, lifestyle habits, and other factors. Based on that information, the insurance company quotes yearly premiums for different types of insurance plans from which you may you select. According to the organization America's Health Insurance Plans, the average annual premium in 2007 for individual plans was $2,613. The average premium for family plans was $5,799. It is important to remember that people typically have to meet a deductible and make copayments for the services and medications they need.

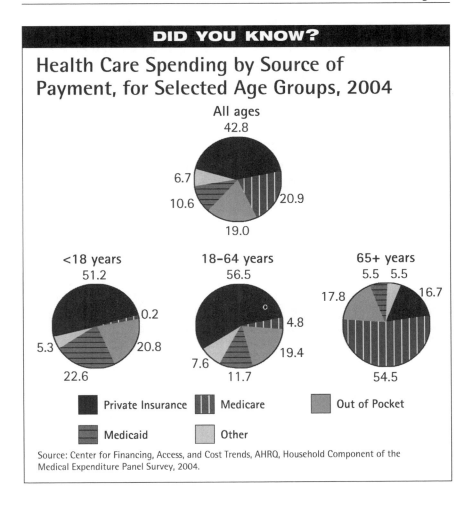

DID YOU KNOW?

Health Care Spending by Source of Payment, for Selected Age Groups, 2004

All ages

<18 years

18–64 years

65+ years

Private Insurance   Medicare   Out of Pocket

Medicaid   Other

Source: Center for Financing, Access, and Cost Trends, AHRQ, Household Component of the Medical Expenditure Panel Survey, 2004.

Signing up for a government-sponsored insurance plan can be difficult. A person or family needs to meet certain income criteria. Each state defines the eligibility criteria. These criteria are based on the U.S. Department of Health and Human Service's Federal Poverty Guidelines. In 2008, a one-person household would need to earn $10,400 or less to be considered in poverty. A family of four would have to earn $21,200 or less to be considered in poverty. States can use the federal guidelines or adjust them based on the cost of living. For example, the income eligibility requirement in Connecticut is 185 percent of the Federal Poverty Guidelines. In this case, a household of one would require an income of $19,240 or less to qualify for Medicaid. For a family of four, the income requirement is $39,220 or less.

Among working adults, the most common way to obtain health insurance is through an employer. Many employers offer health insurance benefits. Some companies pay for this completely. Most companies require employees to pay part of the premium, and they supplement the rest. Companies spend a great deal of money to insure employees. In a 2007 report by the Kaiser Family Foundation, researchers found the average annual cost of health insurance through an employer is $4,497. This is single coverage, meaning only the employee is insured. It costs $12,106 to insure the employee and his or her family. The research also found that employers covered 84 percent of the yearly premium for every employee who signed up for single coverage. Employers paid 72 percent of the yearly premium for every employee who elected to have family coverage.

EMPLOYER DISCRIMINATION AGAINST SMOKERS

The CDC estimates that smokers have $1,623 in excess medical expenses. The North Carolina Department of Health and Human Services reports that each employee who smokes costs an employer $1,429 per year in additional health-care costs.

Employers obviously have financial incentives to monitor the health of their employees. The more insurance claims filed by employees, the higher the premiums will become. Because employers cover most of the premiums, they are essentially being punished for the habits of their employees. When it comes to employer-sponsored insurance, insurance companies evaluate the collective risk, instead of an individual's risk.

Many companies are now trying to find ways to reduce their health insurance costs. For example, a 2006 article in *USA Today* discussed how several companies started having smokers pay a higher percentage of their health insurance premiums. Companies such as Pepsi and General Mills began charging smokers an additional $20 to $50 a month for health insurance. A 2008 story in the *Evansville Courier Press* reported that Whirlpool suspended 39 employees who lied about their smoking habits on insurance forms. The company makes smokers pay an additional $500 a year for their health insurance. Many companies will also make employees pay for a greater share of their health insurance if any family members smoke.

Another tactic companies are starting to use is refusing to hire smokers. Union Pacific, a railroad company, stopped hiring smokers in 2004. In states where it is legal to do so, employers will imme-diately reject job applicants who smoke. Not all states allow this, because it is often considered discrimination.

Many companies are starting to offer smoking-cessation programs. Smokers are given the option of engaging in wellness programs or going through a program to help them quit smoking. Smokers who fail to participate in these must pay a higher percentage of their health insurance premium.

Insurance companies are also starting to cover the cost of smok-ing cessation programs. Nonsmokers cost less to insure than smokers. Thus, insurers would rather pay for members to quit smoking instead of paying smoking-related medical bills.

See also: Cost of Smoking; Therapies for Quitting

FURTHER READING

Pitcher, Timothy J. *How to Make Sense of Health Insurance in America: The Consumer Choice Edition.* Oxford, U.K.: Trafford Publishing, 2006.

■ LAWS AGAINST SMOKING

See: Government and Tobacco; Secondhand Smoke

■ MEDIA AND SMOKING, THE

Early forms of mass media helped popularize cigarettes. Today, films still tend to make smoking seem glamorous. The news media, however, have proven to be more of a problem for tobacco companies, reveal-ing health problems related to smoking and embarrassing corporate secrets.

SHAPING THE PUBLIC'S PERCEPTION

Americans initially had a negative impression of cigarette smoking, partly because of a publicity photograph that was widely reprinted. In 1851, a photograph of a Spanish dancer named Lola Montez showed her with a cigarette. Although Montez was actually a young Irish woman, she was seen as foreign and even exotic. She later became the mistress of the king of Bavaria. Montez's photo planted the idea that smoking was something done by foreigners—and immoral women. This image was reinforced when the opera *Carmen* came to the United States in 1878. In the days before films and television, opera was a popular form of entertainment. *Carmen* was set in a Spanish cigarette factory. The heroine smoked and seduced young men, reinforcing the impression given by Montez.

Harper's Weekly, the national newspaper/magazine of the time, devoted a fair amount of space to satirizing smoking and smokers. An Internet site devoted to the magazine offers an interesting series of articles entitled "Coffin Nails: The Tobacco Controversy in the 19th Century." The initial view in *Harper's* was that people who rolled their own cigarettes were either up to no good or had too much time on their hands.

Cigarette smoking was not considered manly until soldiers in the Spanish-American War brought the habit home in the late 1890s. Even then, as the *Harper's* web site points out, military officials tried to discourage soldiers and sailors from smoking.

By 1907, a whole new medium had appeared—silent films. Most were crude and relied on stereotypes. Country folk smoked pipes, solid citizens smoked cigars, poorer city dwellers and citified dandies smoked cigarettes. As for women, at first only naughty women smoked.

By the 1920s, however, more women smoked, and smoking on-screen became less naughty and more sophisticated. During this era, national brands were establishing themselves in the cigarette market. Companies used signs, billboards, and newspaper ads to push such slogans as "I'd walk a mile for a Camel!"

In 1929, Lucky Strike, a company that was trying to recruit female smokers, hired several young women to light up and smoke during New York's famous Easter Parade. The images of the attractive women challenging a stuffy society event appeared in newspapers all over the country, tying in perfectly with the advertising campaign for Luckies.

SMOKING ON THE BIG AND SMALL SCREENS

In the 1930s, talking pictures replaced the silent films. Increasingly, characters in these films smoked, and many female stars posed for glamour photos with cigarettes in two-foot-long holders.

In 1942, the film *Now, Voyager* featured one of the great romantic smoking scenes as suave Paul Henreid lit up two cigarettes at once and

Bette Davis took one of them from his lips. In *Casablanca*, Humphrey Bogart perfected his tough but tarnished good-guy character. The image of Bogart with his trench coat, fedora hat, and a cigarette dangling from his lips set the look for movie, and later TV, detectives. These media images were very powerful and resulted in increased smoking. According to American Lung Association statistics, consumption of cigarettes nearly doubled during World War II, rising from 181.9 billion in 1940 to 340.6 billion in 1945. Part of the increase may have been due to the inclusion of free cigarettes in the rations of servicemen.

By the 1950s, smoking was almost everywhere. Movie stars smoked on screen and endorsed cigarettes in magazine ads. It wasn't just advertised on the new medium of TV, lead characters smoked in television series. Some featured not only smoking detectives but also doctors who smoked. Even the most respected newsman of the era, Edward R. Murrow, smoked while he interviewed newsmakers on TV.

Murrow did not smoke on camera when CBS-TV's *See It Now* presented the first program linking cancer and smoking in 1955. But he didn't quit either, feeling it was already too late. He died of lung cancer in 1965. As more news about the dangers of smoking became public, more stars who smoked began dying. Humphrey Bogart died from cancer of the esophagus in 1957. John Wayne, who played indestructible he-men in more than 150 movies, lost a lung and part of his stomach to cancer in 1963. His last film, *The Shootist*, came out in 1976. It was about a big, indestructible gunfighter who was dying of cancer. Two years later Wayne was dead from stomach cancer.

THE MEDIA AND THE SMOKING CONTROVERSY

Although scientists had been making connections between smoking and serious health conditions since the 1930s, few of these discoveries made their way into the news. Publishers were unwilling to offend tobacco companies, who were major advertisers. The first major print exposure for the health risks of smoking came in a 1952 article in *Reader's Digest* magazine entitled "Cancer by the Carton." In 1964 the **surgeon general,** the nation's highest public health official, issued a report on health dangers from smoking. Cigarette manufacturers fought back with full-page ads in newspapers. Organizations like the Tobacco Industry Research Institute (TIRC), an industry group funded by tobacco companies, hired writers to create articles that confused the issues related to smoking. They then got those stories published in magazines and distributed them as "media coverage" to editors and publishers.

The fight between antismoking forces and the tobacco companies took place with a war of press releases, news stories, and TV commercials. The tobacco side lost heavily in 1971 when Congress banned cigarette advertising from television and radio. But cigarette brand names and logos still appeared on television, thanks to the way tobacco companies sponsored sporting events. In the 1980s, companies also began paying for the placement of their products in films. Cigarette packs and logos began appearing in the background of many films, and stars began smoking. Formerly secret tobacco company documents show that in 1983 Sylvester Stallone actually had a $500,000 deal with the Brown & Williamson tobacco company to smoke their products in five films.

TEENS SPEAK

My First and Last Pack of Cigarettes

Steve is a freshman in college. He hopes to major in theater and does a close-up magic act at a local restaurant.

"I'll never forget the first pack of cigarettes I bought. Finally used my own money. I'd been smoking for a while, bumming cigarettes from my friends. Even then, I was doing the magic. I'd take a butt, make it disappear, and then smoke it myself.

"I tried to copy the way my favorite actors in the movies smoked, or I'd try to do tricks with the smoke. You know, blow smoke rings, the French inhale, stupid stuff.

"Anyway, I finally graduated to buying my own. It was Saturday night, and I was at a party. I met a girl and wanted to impress her. So I kept offering her cigarettes. Every time I did, I had one myself.

"'Hey,' she finally said, 'You must be a pretty heavy smoker.'

That was the problem. I wasn't. I ended up running for the bathroom. It was a toss–up whether I would pass out, or make it to the bowl and throw up.

He laughs. "Either way, I didn't look so cool. It was a while before I could look at a cigarette without getting sick."

ROLE MODELS AND SMOKING

A 2005 study in *Pediatrics* focused on whether exposure to smoking in the movies influenced a juvenile's decision to start smoking. The authors conducted a phone survey with 6,522 juveniles ages 10 to 14. The authors found that the more adolescents are exposed to smoking in movies, the more likely they are to start smoking.

Even in the smallest movie theater, the screen is billboard-sized. When young people see smoking in films, they're seeing a larger-than-life ad.

WHAT IS THE ALLURE?

Smoking scenes in old movies not only record the attitude toward tobacco in past decades but also color popular culture today. The lonesome cowboy rolling his own cigarette by a campfire, the lovers sharing cigarettes, the hero taking a hard drag on a cigarette before embarking on the desperate fight—these images were established in the 1940s, but almost anyone today will recognize them. The same thing happens today. Lois Lane, in *Superman Returns,* smokes throughout the movie. Other movies, such as *Talladega Nights* and *You, Me, and Dupree* contain excessive amounts of smoking, according to the American Medical Association.

The argument can certainly be made that these are only images. But young people, especially teens, are very aware of image. Consider this comment from a young reviewer analyzing films for tobacco content. "The smoking in *Chicago* is consistently portrayed as incredibly sexy and cool," the 16-year-old said. "And how couldn't it be sexy and cool when Catherine Zeta-Jones does it?"

Fact Or Fiction?

So what if the star in a movie lights up? It's all make-believe.

The Facts: The make-believe is especially important for tobacco companies. In 1996, a California-based group of teen researchers working with a local affiliate of the American Lung Association began analyzing films for tobacco use. They discovered that lead characters smoked five times as often as people did in real life, which may explain why many believe that smoking is a widely accepted part of life.

THE DECEPTION

Formerly secret corporate documents reveal that tobacco companies made smoking in the movies a priority. "Smoking is being positioned as an unfashionable, as well as unhealthy, custom," a major executive for Philip Morris, the leading American tobacco company, told his marketing staff in 1983. "We must continue to exploit new opportunities to get cigarettes on screen and into the hands of smokers."

A program run by the Sacramento, California, chapter of the American Lung Association finds the industry continuing those activities 20 years later. Watching the top films of 2003, reviewers 14 to 22 years old used a standardized form to analyze scenes where tobacco appeared. They found that 80 percent of the PG-13 films—movies that teens can attend alone—featured smoking and tobacco. Further, the reviewers found pro-tobacco messages in 74 percent of those films.

Filmgoers don't expect commercials in the middle of a film. Antismoking activists are concerned that smoking scenes don't come with the health warnings that appear on cigarette packs and regular advertising.

Q & A

Question: My friend is probably the prettiest girl in seventh grade. But she does everything her favorite movie star does. Well, this movie star smoked up a storm in her last movie, so now my friend is trying to do the same. How can I convince her this isn't a good idea?

Answer: Explain to your friend that imitation is not the sincerest—or healthiest—form of flattery. In a 2006 report from the National Institute of Drug Abuse, researchers found evidence that adolescents are more vulnerable to nicotine addiction. Even occasional smoking can lead to becoming hooked on nicotine. Apparently, young people's developing brains are much more sensitive to nicotine. Girls have been known to show signs of addiction after only three weeks of occasional smoking. If your friend doesn't stop quickly, she may end up smoking for years.

NEGATIVE STORIES ABOUT SMOKING

While tobacco companies encourage media exposure that shows smoking in a positive light, they're less eager about exposure that has negative implications.

When the magazine *Mother Jones* ran a strong antismoking story, tobacco companies withheld advertising for five years.

Philip Morris sued ABC-TV for $10 billion over a 1994 news-magazine segment that accused tobacco companies of manipulating **nicotine** in cigarettes. The case was settled out of court with the TV network apologizing. In 1995, a similar case had a very different ending. Jeffrey Wigand, a former head of research for Brown & Williamson, agreed to discuss health problems involved with cigarettes and nicotine on CBS-TV's *60 Minutes*.

Before the Wigand interview could air, CBS lawyers and executives killed the story. They feared being sued for $15 billion by Brown & Williamson.

Wigand went on to testify in a class-action lawsuit against the tobacco companies. What he said in the courtroom was essentially what he told *60 Minutes*. The *Wall Street Journal* covered the story— and the tobacco company's attempts to discredit Wigand. In the end, Wigand's interview appeared on a 1996 *60 Minutes* segment. Brown & Williamson's attempts to silence him ironically gave his interview greater publicity. In fact, the story moved beyond the news media to Hollywood. A major motion picture about the whole episode, *The Insider*, enjoyed great success and was nominated for best picture at the 2000 Oscar Awards.

MEDIA POWER

The Jeffrey Wigand incident is just one in a long relationship between tobacco companies and the media. Corporations not only used the media for advertising and publicity but also exerted influence on both entertainment and news. The most troubling aspect of Wigand's story is that it reveals the great reach tobacco companies have in determining what does and doesn't come before the American public.

See also: Advertising and Smoking; Women and Smoking

FURTHER READING
Gately, Iain. *Tobacco*. New York: Grove Press, 2002.

Malaspina, Ann. *False Images, Deadly Promises: Smoking and the Media.* Broomall, Pa.: Mason Crest, 2008.

■ MEDICATIONS AND SMOKING

To ensure that medications do not interact dangerously with chemicals normally found in the human body, prescription drugs undergo years of safety testing before they are allowed on the market. Even then, warnings about drug interactions appear on the packaging of both prescription and over the counter medications.

Cigarette smoke contains some 4,000 chemicals, and the act of smoking brings these chemicals into the body. The most active substance is **nicotine,** which initiates numerous activities both in the brain and the body. That activity can change when nicotine is combined with prescription medications. Interactions might cause a medicine to be less effective, or they can increase the action of a drug. Another result could be an unexpected side effect.

Fact Or Fiction?

Smoking a cigarette can't affect any medication I take.

The Facts: Years ago, perhaps, a cigarette was just tobacco wrapped in paper. Today, with up to 600 ingredients being added to the tobacco, cigarette smoke is a combination of more than 4,000 chemicals, including nicotine, a drug that affects both the brain and the body. If you're taking medications—especially new medications—you should check with your doctor and pharmacist.

NICOTINE AND MEDICINE

As nicotine enters the body, it causes a series of direct reactions in various organs. These reactions counteract the effects of certain drugs.

Theophylline, for example, is a medicine that opens the passages that channel air into the lungs. Nicotine causes these air passages to constrict, or tighten up, countering the effect of the drug. Since theophylline is part of many medications for asthma, patients can have trouble breathing. In fact, anyone taking an asthma medication should examine the instructions that accompany the prescription. Most contain warnings about smoking while taking it. People with asthma or any breathing difficulty are usually urged to give up smoking and avoid tobacco smoke.

Another direct effect of nicotine is a constriction, or narrowing, of blood vessels in the body, which causes a sharp rise in blood pressure. If a patient is diagnosed with hypertension (high blood pressure) or is already on medication for that condition, his or her smoking habits must be discussed with the doctor. The prescription dose may need to be altered.

Nicotine also makes the heart beat faster. Certain medicines prescribed for heart disease may have more difficulty controlling cardiac problems if the patient smokes.

When prescribing medication, a physician expects a certain dosage of the substance to remain in the body for a specific amount of time. That's why some pills are taken once per day, while other drugs require multiple doses during the day. Enzymes released from the liver help to break down medications in the bloodstream. Enzymes are body chemicals that trigger chemical reactions, such as the breakdown of food into substances the body can use and wastes that will be excreted. Drug companies calculate their dosages based on the rate of breakdown and excretion for a medicine by the amount of enzymes normally found in the body.

However, the nicotine in cigarette smoke stimulates the liver to produce additional amounts of certain enzymes. These extra enzymes can eliminate medicine in the blood too quickly, reducing the effectiveness of the prescription.

What kinds of drugs are affected? Actually, smoking has been shown to reduce the effectiveness of a wide range of medicines. These include anticoagulant drugs that thin the blood like Heparin, and pain medications like Talwin and Darvon. Some types of antianxiety drugs may be affected, like Librium and Valium. Nicotine also reduces the effects of antipsychotic drugs such as chlorpromazine, clozapine, and olanzapine. Certain antidepressant drugs have a reduced effect as well because stimulants like nicotine affect the heart rate.

Smoking also has effects on insulin production by the pancreas, an important consideration for people with diabetes. Nicotine is also mentioned in relation to Viagra, although not as an interaction. Smoking and other types of nicotine use have been linked to erectile dysfunction. This condition may be due to poor blood circulation and could actually be a warning of impending cardio-vascular disease. One can usually reverse the condition by stopping smoking.

MIXING NICOTINE WITH NICOTINE

Perhaps the most obvious danger comes from mixing nicotine with nicotine. Smokers attempting to quit may use both over-the-counter and prescription nicotine replacement therapies—the patch, gum, loz-enges, or an inhaled nicotine spray. Instructions for the use of these products make it clear that users cannot smoke while using these treatments.

Each nicotine replacement therapy method depends on deliver-ing a measured dose of nicotine to blunt cravings as the user quits. Smoking introduces additional nicotine into the system, perhaps more nicotine than the body can handle. Nicotine is, after all, a poison. If nicotine levels in the body are too high, toxic reactions occur. Symptoms of nicotine overdose include cold sweat, dizziness, feeling sick to the stomach, rapid heartbeat, weakness, drooling, confusion, and even fainting. If such symptoms occur, a doctor should be called immediately.

Talk to your doctor

In the past, most Americans went to a family doctor who had an intimate knowledge of their medical history. Today many people may have a variety of physicians who may not be aware of a patient's entire health picture.

It becomes the patient's responsibility to keep all of his or her doc-tors updated on prescriptions presently being taken as well as allergies and lifestyle choices. Patients should alert their doctors to smoking and other habits so that they can prescribe appropriate medicines and dosages. A discussion with a doctor or pharmacist about prescriptions can help to avoid some unpleasant side effects.

RECENT RESEARCH REVEALS A PUZZLE

In 2002, scientists at the Scripps Research Institute in California stud-ied the way nicotine breaks down in the human body. They discovered that one of the products of that breakdown, a compound called nornic-otine, does considerably more than anyone had previously thought.

Nornicotine appears naturally in tobacco and tobacco smoke. Unlike nicotine, which breaks down quickly, nornicotine remains in the bloodstream.

Nicotine in the body acts like a **neurotransmitter,** a chemical which helps to deliver messages along nerves, creating certain responses in the brain and in other organs. Nornicotine acts as a **catalyst,** a substance that causes chemical reactions to occur. Previously, scientists believed that only enzymes performed this function in the human body. Now they have found that nornicotine interacts in important bodily reactions like turning the sugar glucose into energy or affecting medications. Tests have determined that nornicotine reacts with prescription steroids like cortisone and prednisone, possibly making them more toxic. There may also be reactions with antibiotics.

Scientists have found that it is possible that nornicotine may be able to delay the onset of Alzheimer's disease. However, nornicotine is both very addictive and toxic, making it a difficult chemical to use as a treatment.

Tests on animals and humans are currently underway to see what potential adverse effects may exist. But another tobacco chemical which had been little known and considered to be a bystander in the body has certainly shown surprises—both dangerous and potentially beneficial.

Q & A

Question: My friend has been a smoker for months, but he's managed to keep it a secret from his family and almost everyone else. The thing is, he's going to a new doctor who says he's depressed and needs medicine. Shouldn't my friend come clean and tell the doctor about his smoking?

Answer: Medicines for depression may not work as well on a smoker as a nonsmoker. Also, smoking while on these medications can pose a serious risk to a person's heart. Explain these points to your friend and encourage him to discuss all aspects of his health with his new doctor.

See also: Alcohol and Tobacco Use; Drugs and Tobacco Use

FURTHER READING

American Medical Association. *American Medical Association Family Medical Guide, 4th Edition.* Hoboken, N.J.: Wiley, 2004.

Goldmann, David R., ed. *American College of Physicians Complete Home Medical Guide.* New York: DK Publishing, 2003.

◼ MOUTH AND SMOKING, THE

The mouth is a major gateway to the body, providing access to the stomach and the lungs and permitting human speech. Besides letting words out, the mouth permits entry of food and air (many people breath by mouth, especially when they are exerting themselves).

Of course, the mouth also allows entry to germs, pollen, and pollutants, so it also must serve as one of the first lines of defense for the body. Many people consider saliva to be "mouth juice," something to keep the lips and tongue moist. Saliva is actually a mixture of mucus and enzymes, substances which trigger chemical changes (such as breaking down proteins, which helps to destroy bacteria in the mouth). Saliva traps bacteria and rinses and cleans the mouth.

No matter how people use tobacco—whether they smoke, chew, or dip snuff or smokeless tobacco—the mouth is always affected. Continuous exposure to cigarette smoke makes the mouth the secondary deposit site for nicotine, tar, and the numerous chemicals that enter the body with every puff.

When people discuss smoking, the long-term problems get the most attention—risks of lung cancer, heart attack, and stroke. Some consequences of tobacco use come earlier, however. The mouth must deal with damage on a daily basis, and that damage results in some of the most notable changes in the body. It can also lead to disfigurement.

Fact Or Fiction?

People make a lot of fuss over a little bad breath.

The Facts: Smoker's breath is the least of the mouth problems smokers face. Smokers can lose teeth and risk losing parts of their jawbones, tongues, and even their faces from oral cancers.

GUM DISEASE

People rarely pay much attention to their teeth unless they hurt. However, teeth are pretty amazing. With the help of powerful muscles in the jaw, teeth can exert pressure as high as 7,000 pounds per square inch. Usually, that's more than enough to handle the jobs of cutting, tearing, and chewing food. Teeth help in the production of sounds for speech as well. They also help define the shape of the face. Only about one-third of the tooth—the crown—is visible. The rest is anchored solidly in the flesh of the gums.

Just as chemicals in cigarette smoke cause problems for the tissues in the lungs, smoke causes damage to the gums in the mouth. Smokers are much more likely to have problems with **calculus**, not the math, but the hardened dental plaque that forms on the lower sections of teeth and under the gums. Plaque is a sticky combination of mucus, bacteria, and tiny food particles. As the plaque hardens, bacteria in the calculus attack the tissues of the gums, creating pockets that fill with more bacteria, which in turn attack more gum tissue. The skin of the gums begins to pull away from the teeth. If the condition continues, it can lead to a loss of bone, connective tissue—and teeth.

In the early 1900s, many people over the age of 60 had no teeth. They lost them as a result of decay or gum disease. With modern dentistry people over 60 are more likely to have all their teeth. The exceptions are smokers, whose gums are often swollen and receding from the teeth. The American Academy of Periodontology, the branch of dentistry concerned with gum health, warns that smoking accelerates the progress of gum disease.

Smokers' teeth need considerable dental work. To remove calculus, the dentist must physically scrape the teeth, including the area below the gumline. Because smokers often use breath mints, and sugar causes considerable tooth decay, dental visits are usually more painful for smokers and treatments less effective. One of the effects of smoking is a reduction of oxygen in the blood. With less oxygen and fewer nutrients, gum tissues heal more slowly and are more prone to infection.

According to a 2000 study by the Centers for Disease Control and Prevention (CDC), smokers are four times more likely than nonsmokers to suffer from gum disease. Those who smoke more than a pack and a half per day are six times more likely to face infection.

Cigarette smoke isn't the only product that irritates the gums. Smokeless tobacco also irritates gum tissues. In fact, because a pinch of snuff is held between the lip and gum, the effect is often concentrated in that section of the mouth. The gums can start receding deeply. Smokeless tobacco also causes open sores in the mouth and gums and can cause *leukoplakia*, precancerous growths in the mouth.

Disturbing new research

Recent dental research not only links smoking to gum disease but also suggests that the combination of smoking and gum disease can lead to other ailments. A 2001 study reported in the *Journal of Periodontology* suggests that chemicals in tobacco smoke may create a favorable environment for bacteria that cause gum disease. Ongoing research at the University of Manitoba Dental School focuses on several issues related to tobacco and gum disease, including whether smoking causes the release of enzymes that inflame and harm gum tissues.

Researchers think that gum disease bacteria release toxins that travel through the bloodstream. These toxins could be responsible for the inflammation in blood vessels that is connected with cardiovascular disease. Some of these chemical agents may also contribute to creating the blood clots that cause heart attacks and stroke. In 2002, the *Journal of the American Dental Association* examined nine studies that linked gum disease with heart disease. Although the reviewers found that the evidence was not strong enough to make a definite connection, research continues.

Q & A

Question: I met this really great person of the opposite sex, funny, smart—and a smoker. I didn't mind the cigarettes coming out, but when we said good night, it was like kissing a full ashtray! How can I let an otherwise great person know about this problem?

Answer: If you don't speak up, the problem will always be there. If you like your new friend, you'll have to discuss it. There's definitely room for diplomacy, however. The next time the cigarettes come out, you may want to turn the conversation to smoking. It's one way to learn about the other person. You don't have to be insulting or preachy. Maybe you'll find out why the other person began the habit.

You may even discover that your friend is tired of smoking. Perhaps you can help him or her quit. One thing is for sure: you'll never get to know a person better than when they're going through withdrawal.

STAINING AND LOSS OF TEETH

In 1624, the Dutch painter Rembrandt van Rijn painted a group of soldiers. Since the 1800s, the group portrait has been called "The Night Watch," because the soldiers seem to be marching in darkness. When the painting was cleaned in 1946, the restorers discovered that the soldiers were not on a night march after all. Over the centuries, soot and smoke had darkened the varnish protecting the painting, turning it brown—and turning day into night.

Inside your mouth, smoking does a similar job—and much more quickly. When tar, the solid particles in tobacco smoke that collect in the lungs, mixes with saliva in the mouth, it coats the teeth. The effect is much like brushing a liquid stain onto wood. Every time a smoker lights up, a new coat is applied. Brushing and flossing help to minimize staining, but few people brush after every cigarette.

After a few years of smoking, tobacco stains the outside of the teeth. A dentist can clean off the discoloration. With time, however, stains become established in microscopic cracks in the tooth enamel, the outer covering of the tooth. The discoloration becomes harder to remove and can become permanent. Teeth take on a brownish color, and flat surfaces where the tar is able to accumulate can even become black. Teeth can also show increased wear on their biting surfaces.

Although staining is unattractive, it doesn't cause serious harm to the teeth. Gum disease, however, does. As the gums recede, they expose the roots of the teeth. The bacteria in the gum pockets don't just attack the tissue of the gums, they weaken the bone and the connective tissue that holds the teeth in place.

The result is painful teeth. According to a study by Tufts University in Boston, those who smoke a pack a day can expect to lose 2.9 teeth after 10 years of smoking. During the same 10 years, nonsmokers will lose 1.3 teeth. At that rate, a person who started smoking at age 18 and smoked a pack per day would lose four to five teeth by age 35.

The Tufts researchers also found that smokers who quit lost fewer teeth. However, ex-smokers still lost more teeth than nonsmokers.

Replacing lost teeth or trying to stabilize loose ones is expensive. Unreplaced teeth have a definite effect on one's appearance—consider how someone's smile would look with gaps in it. Lost teeth may also change the shape of the face.

BAD BREATH

Visit a smoker's house and you'll probably notice a sharp, hard-to-miss smell. The distinctive odor of cigarette smoke sinks into furniture upholstery, clothing, even hair and skin. And, if you've ever been face-to-face with a smoker, you also know that smoking also affects the breath.

Unless a smoker brushes after every cigarette, the residue of cigarette smoke remains on the breath, including the tar particles that stain the teeth. But that's just the tip of the iceberg. Saliva washes away and neutralizes bacteria in the mouth. Smoking dries oral tissues, leaving a smoker with a mouthful of germs and their waste products. The result is not a pretty smell.

Add in the fact that gum disease has its own distinctive aroma and you have three sources for offensive odors. Smoking may look cool on a movie screen, but up close and personal, it might be less enjoyable.

A VERY VISIBLE PROBLEM

Much of the damage that smoking does to a person—cancer, for instance, or heart and lung disease—takes place deep within the body over many years. What smoking does to the mouth, however, happens more quickly, and the results are more public. Stained teeth, bad breath, or a gap-toothed smile are hard to ignore. These conditions definitely affect the impression a person makes.

See also: Alcohol and Tobacco Use; Cosmetic Effects of Smoking; Drugs and Tobacco Use

FURTHER READING

Goldmann, David R., ed. *American College of Physicians Complete Home Medical Guide.* New York: DK Publishing, 2003.

Hyde, Margaret O., and John F. Setevo, M.P. *Smoking 101: An Overview for Teens.* Minneapolis: Twenty-first Century Books, 2006.

■ PEER PRESSURE AND SMOKING

Peer pressure is the influence that people your age exert on your behavior, values, habits, and beliefs. People of all ages—from toddlers to adults—encounter peer pressure. However, peer pressure seems to have the most impact on teenagers. It can affect what teens wear, what music they listen to, the shows they watch on television, whether they play or follow sports (and which ones), and what habits they share. Put simply, the people around a young person can affect whether he or she begins smoking. According to the 1994 surgeon general's report, "Preventing Tobacco Use Among Young People," peers have the greatest effect on whether a young person tries cigarettes and continues to experiment with tobacco.

Although peer pressure can come from an older sibling, in most cases, it involves friends and acquaintances, often in a school setting. Everyone has gone through the experience of being the "new kid in school," whether it's a move to a new town or a transition from elementary to middle school or high school. Even those coming to a new school with a group of friends may experience the sensation of being alone in a crowd or feel as if they're being scrutinized. They may find themselves wondering, "Am I going to fit in around here? *Where* am I going to fit in around here?" Ironically, that hard-eyed crowd of strangers around you is actually composed of people stressing over what kind of impression *they* are making.

In the movies, peer pressure is often dramatic. Powerful strangers or near-strangers demand that the hero go along with something that is wrong. Very rarely in real life do complete strangers ask someone to do something illegal or risky.

Peer pressure is often a series of small steps, sometimes not very clear-cut, involving close friends. It might start with a friend asking you to hold his pack of cigarettes while he's playing basketball. Maybe the next time he lights up, he'll offer you one. Perhaps when he's upset about some problem, you'll notice how he visibly calms down after a couple of puffs. Sometime when you're stressed out about something, he offers you a cigarette.

Fact Or Fiction?

All that stuff about 'peer pressure' and smoking is blown way out of proportion.

The Facts: Peer pressure is an important issue in determining when and how young people try their first cigarettes. In a 2005 study in *Pediatrics*, the authors found that adolescents with friends who smoke are at least three times more likely to smoke than adolescents without friends who smoke.

WHAT DO THE NUMBERS SAY?

Public health officials are concerned about the decisions teens might make concerning their safety and wellness. Every two years, thousands of students register their opinions on dangerous activities through the Centers for Disease Control and Prevention's Youth Risk Behavior Surveillance System. The National Center for Addiction and Substance Abuse gathers similar information through its annual survey, "Monitoring the Future." Philip Morris, the giant tobacco firm, also surveyed students in 2007 for its Youth Smoking and Prevention Teenage Attitudes and Behavior Study.

One of the questions asked in the Phillip Morris survey was why the person currently smokes. Only 17 percent of those age 11 through 17 said it was because their friends smoke. The most common reason given was, "It helps me relax," followed by "I like it," and "Out of habit." Even though peer pressure is not one of the top reasons for smoking, smokers are more likely to have friends who smoke. Among those who reported smoking, 28.1 percent said their three to four closest friends also smoked. Only 10.8 percent of youth reported smoking when one or two of their closest friends also smoked.

Another study followed slightly older smokers—278 males and 443 females starting their senior year of high school—and continued for five years. Researchers tried to evaluate factors that may have impacted the subjects' decisions to smoke. The results were published in 2002 in the journal *Nicotine and Tobacco Research*. The researchers concentrated on a range of issues that may have affected decisions about smoking: teens' beliefs on the subject, rebellious feelings, attitudes about risky behaviors, the attitude of parents, and peer pressure.

The study found that while peer pressure might encourage young people to start smoking, it could also play a part in getting a smoker to stop. After five years, 12 percent of the males and 17 percent of the females reported that they had quit smoking and had not smoked in a year. The males reported more difficulty in resisting pressure from friends to smoke. Females found it easier to quit if their parents had disapproved of their high school smoking and if their old high school friends didn't smoke.

In a 2008 study in *The Journal of Genetic Psychology*, the authors took a very interesting approach to examining peer pressure and smoking. They looked at identical twins to see how friendships may influence smoking. For each pair of twins, one smoked and the other did not. The findings indicated that friends influenced smoking behavior. Peer pressure did play a role; however, other factors were present as well. Reasons included wanting an image change and engaging in rebellious behavior.

SELF-FULFILLING EXPECTATIONS?

Surveys about smoking also give ample evidence that young people's perceptions don't always match reality. As both the surgeon general's report on teen smoking and a 1995 study in the *New England Journal of Medicine* show, young people, especially smokers, consistently overestimate the percentage of people who smoke. Partly, this is due to the media. Since 1996, a group of young reviewers working with the American Lung Association of Sacramento–Emigrant Trails in California has monitored smoking content in movies. In some years, the viewers found that the ratio of smoking lead characters to non-smokers was five times greater than in real life. Advertising, too, creates an image of a world in which "everybody" smokes.

When you watch a teen movie, you can expect to see certain types—the popular kids, jocks, regular kids, brains, nonconformists, and burnouts. A 2001 study published in the *Journal of Pediatric Psychology* indicated that teens in real life tend to think in terms of the same stereotypes, and to live up—or down—to the expected image.

The researchers interviewed 250 students, classifying them by types. When asked to discuss their friends, the teens made the same assessments. When it came to health choices like smoking, the people considered nonconformists and burnouts made the riskiest decisions.

DEALING WITH PEER PRESSURE

One respondent to the Philip Morris youth study compared peer pressure to being in a group and suddenly being caught in a spotlight. Like most moments in the spotlight, the best preparation is rehearsal. Unfortunately, there is no set speech that will remove the pressure. The teenage years are a time when people learn to live in the larger world. They have to learn how to make choices and live with them—how to be an individual.

The family connection will always be important, however, and so will the values parents and children share. Part of preparation for life is learning to defend those values. Organizations as widely separated as Philip Morris and the federal government's Substance Abuse and Mental Health Services Administration (SAMHSA) stress the importance of parents working with their children to deal with peer pressure. Like many other youth advocates, they suggest role-playing to illustrate situations that place young people under pressure and to teach them how to think on their feet and respond to these situations.

The consensus is that the earlier families start working together on responses to peer pressure, the more confidently a young person can face the problem. Teens with low self-esteem, who need a lot of reassurance from others, are more likely to be influenced by peer pressure.

Role-playing can teach one how to reject a suggestion without rejecting the friend who makes it. It also lets young people develop answers that match their personalities.

Working with parents on a problem is a great way to keep the lines of communication open. Try to discuss problems you see classmates dealing with and express your own concerns. If your family situation doesn't allow for this kind of communication, you can still talk to someone you respect—a teacher, school counselor, or religious leader perhaps. You can also find help from community or youth groups, peer counselors, or friends. Often when a person is feeling pressured, having just one other person join in on his or her side can make a crucial difference.

If you have younger brothers or sisters, be aware that you can be a positive role model. Talk with your younger siblings about peer pressure. For example, when you say, "When I was your age," it's a lot closer in time than when your parents say it. The sooner you discuss and role play about the problem with kid brothers or sisters, the more aware—and prepared—all the members of your family will be when it comes to dealing with peer pressure.

Q & A

Question: How can I say "no" to my friends and still be part of the group?

Answer: Keep things light and in your usual tone. If you've got an excuse like an allergy, feel free to use it. Don't turn the offer of a cigarette into an argument or a sermon.

After all, if they're really your friends, they should cut you some slack. The members of your group aren't all baseball or basketball fans, are they? There should be room for both smokers and nonsmokers.

If the people you hang out with are insistent that you smoke along with them, you'll have to ask the question: Are they really your friends?

See also: Advertising and Smoking; Media and Smoking, The

FURTHER READING

Aronson, Virginia. *How to Say No.* Philadelphia: Chelsea House, 2000.

McLeod Humphrey, Sandra. *Hot Issues, Cool Choices: Facing Bullies, Peer Pressure, Popularity, and Put-downs.* Amherst, N.Y.: Prometheus Books, 2007.

■ QUITTING, THERAPIES FOR

Smoking is an addiction, a very difficult behavior to change. Many people attempt to overcome smoking by going "cold turkey," using willpower to quit. The failure rate for this method is high. Others use therapies involving prescription or over-the-counter medications to help decrease **cravings** for nicotine during the quitting period. Still other people rely on psychological treatment to control their smoking behavior.

TEENS SPEAK

How I Learned to Quit Smoking

Karen is a 17-year-old high school senior. When she's not in class, she works for a political candidate in her town.

"I started smoking because of my uncle. To me, he was the coolest guy in the world. He worked at the airport, servicing jet engines. In our blue-collar neighborhood that was a really good job.

"Our families were always getting together for barbecues, stuff like that. I remember him with a bottle of beer in one hand and a cigarette at his lips—that was pretty much the way things were in my family. Everybody smoked—my mom and dad, my aunts and uncles, most of my older cousins too. It wasn't all that hard to start picking up cigarettes myself."

Karen stares down at the floor. "Then Uncle Mike got sick. In a year, he went from looking like one of those guys in comic books to a stick.

"I remember him coming home from the hospital—probably the last time he got out. He was hanging on to my aunt's arm. With every step he took, he looked as if he were moving about a ton and a half.

"I stopped smoking the day he died. Don't ask me if it was because I was sad or because I was scared. I just never—*ever*—wanted to look like that."

AVERSION THERAPY

Aversion therapy is based on the idea that implanting an unpleasant sensation or experience will deter a person from following a particular course of action. He or she might start to smoke, for instance, because it's a habit or because the act of smoking gives pleasure. Aversion therapy attempts to replace that pleasant experience with an unpleasant one.

The unpleasant stimulus can be an electric shock. A trained operator tapes electrodes to the smoker's forearms. After testing, whenever the smoker goes to light up, the operator administers as powerful a jolt as the patient can stand. Because of the possibility for physical harm, this treatment should be administered by a licensed clinician.

The patient can also try rapid smoking—consuming two cigarettes as rapidly as possible or taking a deep puff every six seconds. The aim of this technique is to take in enough nicotine to make the smoker ill. Still another form of aversion therapy involves smoking after taking chemical or herbal preparations which, when combined with cigarette smoke, create a disagreeable taste.

Repeating such unpleasant experiences will implant an idea in the brain: "Smoking hurts! Smoking makes me sick! Smoking tastes terrible!" Instead of relying solely on willpower to resist a craving, aversion therapy patients also have a powerful gut reaction.

The Schick Smoking Program, developed at the Schick Shadel Hospital in Seattle, Washington, uses both electrical shocks and fast-puff smoking, along with counseling, to help people stop smoking. The program has been offered as a commercial smoking cessation treatment in clinics around the United States since 1972, with more than 100,000 clients using the treatment.

The Schick program claims a high success rate of more than 50 percent. Half of its patients are smoke-free a year after treatment. As with many commercial smoking cessation programs, however, success statistics are the result of in-house studies rather than unbiased independent research. Aversion therapy is not a popular option. The necessary unpleasantness of the treatment is not consumer-friendly. For safety's sake, this therapy should only be tried with a trained health-care professional.

OPERANT STRATEGIES

Operant strategies are treatments that help to restructure thoughts and change behavior. They are based on the idea that actions and viewpoints are learned and can be unlearned or modified by acquiring new skills.

To make the changes that will result in an end to smoking, patients must work with therapists to understand the situations that trigger their smoking. They deal with questions like "Who, what, and where?" Do particular people spark an urge to smoke either by creating social pressure or stirring conflict? What places or activities prompt thoughts of smoking?

Through multiple sessions, usually in a group-therapy setting, patients develop new strategies. Some try **reduced smoking**, in which the patient gradually reduces the number of cigarettes smoked to 50 percent of his or her original daily number and then stops completely. The idea is that gradually lowering the nicotine dose reduces withdrawal problems.

Nicotine fading is another operant strategy. The patient switches to lower and lower nicotine brands, again reducing nicotine intake in preparation for stopping completely.

Scheduled smoking uses cues to teach a new behavior. Instead of smoking in response to the usual triggers, the patient smokes on a printed schedule. By adapting to longer time periods between cigarettes, the patient learns how to move away from tobacco. Patients also create coping strategies to manage the urge to smoke.

Contingency management is a strategy of rewards for success in changing behavior and punishments for failing to do so. Some smoking cessation programs offer participants refunds or target payments for staying away from cigarettes for a certain number of days or weeks. Other programs use a machine to measure carbon monoxide in a participant's breath. A low carbon monoxide level in the breath shows that a patient has not been smoking and therefore is entitled to a reward.

Relapse prevention is a strategy that supports a patient's reasons for quitting to help him or her overcome cravings and deal with failures. A patient learns that a lapse is just one cigarette and not a reason to ignore all the progress he or she has made and go back to smoking.

The cognitive/behavioral approach regards smoking as a result of a chain of feelings and actions. It starts with an activating stimulus—a person or situation—that offers a cue to the smoker. For instance, a young man who leaves the house after an argument with his parents may think, "I'll feel a lot less stressed if I have a cigarette."

This might lead to automatic thoughts, thoughts and beliefs about day-to-day life that occur almost without conscious notice. In this case, it might be a flicker of memory about the pleasure a cigarette could offer, making the urge to smoke all the stronger. Facilitating beliefs, thoughts that "give permission" for an action, might follow. In this case, the young man might think, "I can have just one" and then actually light up a cigarette. Various strategies can help the patient avoid the stimulus that sets the chain in motion or use prepared responses to say "no."

Practiced arguments about the reasons for quitting can counteract automatic thoughts and facilitating beliefs. Exercises like deep breathing can help a smoker resist a craving. A patient can also "ride the wave" of a craving. To those unfamiliar with cravings, the urge seems unstoppable, like an onrushing tank. In fact, cravings come as a wave. They grow strong but then recede. Patients can become familiar with their cravings, time them, and learn exactly how long they have to hold out.

This sort of therapy has been popular since the 1990s. In recent years, people have been trying to take the lessons of this treatment and apply them without a therapist. Users may work from a book, a learning program, or even from an interactive web site.

Fact Or Fiction?

All it takes to quit smoking is willpower.

The Facts: Quitting on willpower alone rarely succeeds. According to the National Health Interview Survey of 2000, less than 10 percent of those who tried to stop smoking using the "cold turkey" or self-help methods achieved their goal. In the past, smoking was considered to be merely a bad habit. Today, people know that smoking has a physical addiction—to nicotine—and a psychological side. Smokers have considerably more resources to help them quit than they did even 10 years ago.

Mark Twain, the famous American humorist from the 1800s, is still remembered today as a great novelist—and as a cigar smoker. Among his most often-quoted lines is one on smoking: "Quitting smoking is easy. I've done it thousands of times."

HYPNOSIS

Hypnosis is a state of mind somewhat like sleep in which a person's ability to think consciously is weak, so he or she is open to suggestions. A hypnotic trance represents an altered state of consciousness where directions about changing behavior meet little resistance. Typically, a hypnotherapy session lasts about 50 minutes. The patient spends a half hour or more talking to the hypnotherapist, discussing the condition. For the rest of the time, the hypnotherapist puts the patient into a light trance. The patient will concentrate intently and remain in a receptive mood while suggestions are made to the unconscious mind. The therapist's job is to find all the situations in the patient's life that trigger the unthinking response of smoking. These might be stress, conversation, finishing a meal, or taking a break at work.

The hypnotherapist then suggests alternative reactions to break the habitual response. These might include deep-breathing exercises, thinking about a pleasant subject as a distraction, or perhaps substituting gum for a cigarette. Sometimes the hypnotist will suggest some of the unpleasant aspects of smoking—perhaps the smell or the mess.

Hypnotherapy works well in some cases. A number of hypnotherapists claim success rates of better than 80 or 90 percent. After a single session, patients may find their cravings reduced, helping them get through withdrawal. In other cases, the therapy is ineffective, resulting in a failed attempt to quit. Some researchers have classified the hypnotherapy success rate at 20 percent or below.

QUITLINES

Another option available to smokers is the quitline, which offers over-the-phone counseling. Counselors provide smokers with support and strategies to stop smoking. Some quitlines even help smokers develop their own cessation plan.

Quitline counseling can be either proactive or reactive. In proactive counseling, the quitline calls smokers to offer support. In reactive counseling, the smoker calls the quitline for help in combating the urge to smoke. Because quitlines are always available, smokers know they can rely on help over time, if they need it.

Quitlines are available in all 50 states and receive state and federal funding. Even though they are available to everyone, quitlines are underutilized. In a 2005 report by the North American Quitline Consortium (NAQC), researchers found that fewer than 1 percent of smokers in any state use a quitline. As time passes and more smokers learn about the benefits of quitlines, utilization rates should increase.

Another option gaining popularity is the use of Internet-based smoking cessation programs. In addition to quitlines, states are adding Internet-based resources to help smokers kick the habit. The major benefit of these Web sites is their convenience; smokers can use the services any time of day or night. Internet-based programs are not intended to be used as the sole source of help, however. They are typically used in conjunction with other cessation therapies.

The effectiveness of these sites is debatable. In a 2006 study in *Nicotine and Tobacco Research,* the authors found that adding an Internet-based intervention did not improve the success rates of smokers trying to quit. However, one study does not conclusively prove whether a program works. More research will be needed. Even if Internet-based interventions do not increase cessation rates, they still provide a valuable service. In a 2007 study in the *American Journal of Health Studies*, researchers found that participants felt the online service was helpful. There were several reasons for this. The site provided useful information, the ability to talk with others in online forums, and convenient access to support.

SUCCESS RATES

A 2008 study in *Nicotine and Tobacco Research* provided evidence that hypnosis is a viable approach to smoking cessation. Almost 300 smokers were enrolled in a smoking cessation study. They were randomly enrolled in either hypnosis treatment or behavioral counseling. All smokers were given a nicotine patch to use. The authors found that after six months, 24 percent of smokers in the hypnosis group were still smoke-free. This is compared to 18 percent of smokers who were in the behavioral counseling groups. After a year, 20 percent of the participants in the hypnosis group were smoke-free, compared to 14 percent in the behavioral counseling group.

When it comes to aversion therapy, the most well-known practitioners are at the Schick Shadel Hospital. In a 1988 study published in the *Journal of Substance Abuse Treatment,* the hospital claimed a one-year success rate between 50 and 60 percent. In a story on various therapies to quit smoking, the British science magazine *New Scientist* offered a success rate as high as 60 percent for some forms of hypnosis and 25 percent for aversion therapy. However, some sources report that aversion therapy's effect is negligible. In a 2005 review of aversion therapy in the book *Evidence-Based Respiratory Medicine,* the authors found that aversion therapy was not an effective means of quitting smoking. The odds of quitting were 1.05, meaning smokers who tried aversion therapy were .05 times more likely to quit than those who attempted to stop on their own.

Q & A

Question: I'm really worried that my friend is smoking too much. Can you make someone quit smoking?

Answer: You can't force anyone to stop smoking. You can, however, encourage a friend to think about it. There's no need to preach or harp on the subject. Keep it natural and don't push.

Here's a survey you might want to discuss with your friend. When researchers polled teen smokers, only 5 percent of the kids believed they'd be smoking in five years. When the researchers recently did an eight-year follow-up, 75 percent of the people they'd originally talked with were still smoking.

If you can help friends make it into the 25 percent that quit early, you'll be doing them a big favor.

See also: Addiction, Products to Overcome

FURTHER READING

Brizer, David. *Quitting Smoking for Dummies.* New York: Wiley, 2003.

Carr, Allen. *The Easy Way to Stop Smoking.* New York: Sterling, 2005.

Whetherall, Charles. *Quit: Read This Book and Stop Smoking.* Philadelphia: Running Press Miniature Editions, 2007.

■ RESPIRATORY DISEASES AND SMOKING

Smoking causes and aggravates respiratory disease. The respiratory system involves many delicate mechanisms and numerous safeguards to bring oxygen into the body and expel carbon dioxide. Some structures in the lungs are only one cell thick. It should come as no surprise to find that a habit that involves breathing in smoke would have an effect on the lungs.

Some of the chemicals found in tobacco smoke are carcinogens. Over time, they cause genetic damage that may lead to cancer. Other chemicals in the tar in tobacco smoke create more immediate damage. Several lung conditions have been connected with smoking, such as chronic bronchitis, emphysema, and asthma.

Fact Or Fiction?

If someone is out of breath, it means he or she is out of shape.

The Facts: If a person becomes out of breath after moderate exertion, he or she may need more exercise. Before joining a gym, however, that person should see a doctor. Someone who is often short of breath—especially a smoker—could have serious respiratory problems.

HOW RESPIRATION WORKS

Getting oxygen to the cells deep within your body is a complicated task. Each breath takes air in through the mouth and nose and down the throat, voicebox, and windpipe. Then the airway splits into two passages, the **bronchial tubes,** or bronchi. Progressively tinier tubes, bronchioles, continue to split off, leading to the thin-walled air sacs where gases pass into the bloodstream. These **alveoli**, air-exchange sites, look like bunches of balloons. They expand and contract as inhaled air enters and carbon dioxide leaves.

Like balloons, alveoli are delicate. The walls of these tiny structures are only one cell thick. As oxygen passes through this very fine skin and into microscopic blood vessels, carbon dioxide passes in the opposite direction. Any blockage in the airway between the mouth and nose and the blood vessels in the lungs can quickly become a matter of life and death.

When people encounter smoke—from a fire, bus exhaust, or other pollution—the natural reaction is to cough. For a smoker, however, breathing smoke is an everyday habit. Although the lungs no longer respond to every cigarette puff with a cough, they are still irritated. In fact, they become damaged.

CHRONIC BRONCHITIS

The bronchial tubes, or bronchi, are the gateways to the lungs, and they are heavily defended. Special cells in the lining of the bronchial tubes secrete a sticky substance called mucus to trap intruding bacteria or dust particles. The inner lining of the tubes also has tiny hairlike growths called **cilia**. The cilia work like very small fingers to push the mixture of mucus and debris toward the windpipe, where it will be coughed up and expelled.

Simple bronchitis is an infection of the bronchi. When bacteria or viruses attack the walls of the bronchial tubes, cells become irritated, and the bronchi become inflamed. The walls of these tubes swell, reducing the width of the air passage. To catch invading organisms, extra mucus is secreted. When this mucus is coughed up, it contains cells used by the immune system to kill bacteria. This mucus which is often thick, gathers in the narrowed bronchi, resulting in a blocked air route. The body's response is frequent coughing to clear the blockages away.

Anyone who has suffered from a bad cold or a case of flu has experienced acute bronchitis. The condition can also be caused by allergic reactions, breathing dust, or pollution. The most common cause, however, is smoking.

Chemicals in cigarette smoke irritate the tissues lining the bronchial tubes, causing damage and making them inflamed. The bronchial walls become easily infected, extra mucus is secreted, and coughing begins. If a person coughs up mucus almost daily for three months in two or more years, he or she is considered to have chronic bronchitis.

As the condition persists, repeated swelling thickens and scars the bronchial walls, cutting the size of the airway. Extra mucus collects in the bronchi as the normal coughing response becomes less effective. Mucus not only clogs the airway but also creates a bacteria-laden soup which can cause additional infections.

Damage from chronic bronchitis is irreversible. If smoking continues and the disease progresses, the patient can end up so short of breath that he or she is unable to carry on everyday activities. Chronic bronchitis may also become a complicating factor for diseases within the lungs themselves.

EMPHYSEMA

Emphysema is a medical condition in which the tissue of the lungs becomes damaged, making the transfer of oxygen to the blood vessels less efficient. Normal lung tissue is elastic. It changes size as you breathe in and out. Cigarette smoke damages lung tissue, especially the delicate walls of the alveoli, which lose their stretching ability. Eventually the tiny air sacs tear and merge together. Smoking is the number-one cause of emphysema, accounting for 80 percent to 90 percent of all cases.

Healthy lungs are composed of many alveoli (numbering in the millions). Taken together, the alveoli walls offer 100 square yards of thin tissue through which oxygen passes to the blood. Diseased lungs become distended (larger), the surviving alveoli are also larger, but there is more empty space and much less transfer tissue. Inhaled oxygen is wasted, trapped in these oversized air sacs without transferring into the bloodstream.

As alveoli are destroyed, less oxygen is absorbed by the body. Usually the first sign of emphysema is an inability to catch one's breath. Depending on how much of the lung is destroyed, a victim may not be able to climb even a few flights of stairs or work. Simply breathing becomes a full-time job.

Emphysema may run in families—some people produce less of a body chemical that helps to protect the lungs. Other causes include oily smoke from cooking or pollution, but the major cause is smoking. Countries that have few smokers also have low levels of emphysema. The disease seems to strike 10 to 15 percent of smokers. The organization COPD-International states that men are seven times more likely to be diagnosed with emphysema than women.

Emphysema is also known as "lung rot." People with the disease often die of lung failure or from diseases that affect the lungs like pneumonia or flu.

When chronic bronchitis and emphysema appear together, the condition is known as **Chronic Obstructive Pulmonary Disease**, or COPD. At first, the symptoms begin with a mucus-laden cough after getting out of bed. Then the coughing continues through the day, bringing up increasing amounts of mucus. During the winter, sufferers experience frequent chest infections, coughing up yellow or green mucus. Next comes wheezing from the lungs after coughing, then shortness of breath after exertion, and eventually after mild exertion, and ultimately even at rest. Although doctors can prescribe treatments to ease the symptoms, damage from chronic bronchitis and emphysema is irreversible. If the diagnosis is made early, patients can stop further damage by quitting smoking. Usually, however, the diagnosis is made late, and patients end up disabled.

The National Heart Lung and Blood Institute states that COPD is the fourth leading cause of death in the United States. The disease kills more than 120,000 people each year. Approximately 24 million people have COPD, although only half have officially been diagnosed with it. In the 2004 Surgeon General's Report, authors estimate that in 2001, at least 90 percent of COPD deaths were attributed to smoking.

ASTHMA

Asthma is a condition in which air passages to the lung become rapidly inflamed, causing the airways to narrow. People with asthma suffer from wheezing attacks and breathing difficulties. The disease can range from fairly mild to attacks that threaten the patient's life. No one can predict when attacks will occur, how long they'll last, or how severe they will be. Doctors admit that there is still much to be learned about

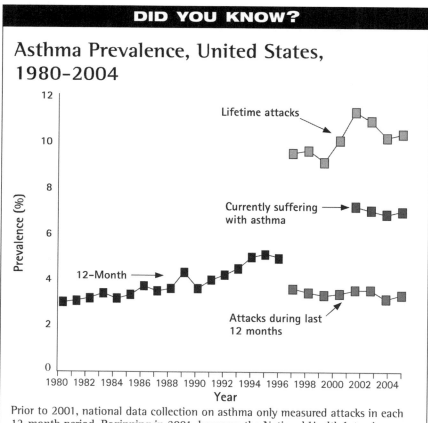

DID YOU KNOW?

Asthma Prevalence, United States, 1980–2004

Prior to 2001, national data collection on asthma only measured attacks in each 12-month period. Beginning in 2001, however, the National Health Interview Survey began to measure three types of prevalence: 1) lifetime asthma attacks; 2) attacks during the last 12 months; and 3) whether or not respondents are currently suffering from the condition.

Source: National Health Interview Survey; National Center for Health Statistics.

the disease, but the known facts are disturbing enough. According to *The Merck Manual,* the number of asthma sufferers increased by 42 percent between 1982 and 1992. That high rate of growth continued through 2001, when the Centers for Disease Control and Prevention found that 20.3 million people were diagnosed with the disease.

Today, an estimated 27.5 million adults report that they have had asthma in their lifetime, according to the Centers for Disease Control. This includes 11.2 million men (10.5 percent of the adult male population) and 16.3 million women (14.3 percent of the adult female population). Approximately 17.3 million adults report that they *currently* suffer from asthma. This includes almost 6 million men (5.6 percent of the adult male population) and 11.3 women (10 percent of the adult female population).

Asthma seems to be an allergic reaction, with the airways of sufferers responding to various triggers with greater sensitivity than those of the general population. Depending on the patient, an attack can come with exposure to pollen, dust mites, animal dander, sulfites (a food preservative), aspirin or other anti-inflammatory drugs, or even cold air. Exercise and stress can sometimes cause an asthma attack. Another major trigger is tobacco smoke.

During an asthma attack, the muscles in the walls of the bronchial tubes spasm, tightening the tubes and cutting the flow of air. Breathing becomes more difficult. Mucus plugs the shrunken air passage, causing coughing and wheezing. Symptoms range from minor discomfort to a life-threatening condition if the path of air is blocked altogether.

Symptoms can include wheezing, a tightness in the chest, and shortness of breath. Sufferers may have a difficult time exhaling and suffer from a persistent cough. Some people have mild asthmatic reactions that can be controlled by staying away from whatever triggers an attack. For most people with asthma, however, there are so many triggers that they must seek treatment.

At present, asthma can be controlled by various drugs in both pill and inhaler form. However, there is no cure. Doctors have many questions: Why do only some people (including some smokers) develop asthma, while others don't? Why do some parts of the country seem to have fewer asthma sufferers than others?

Recent studies show a connection between mothers smoking during pregnancy and asthma in their children. A 2001 study by the University of Southern California not only made this link but also showed that an infant's exposure to secondhand smoke led to the development of asthma in later childhood. A 2004 Finnish study followed 58,841 children from birth to age seven. The study suggested that women who smoked more than 10 cigarettes a day during pregnancy had a 36 percent chance of having a child who developed asthma by age seven. Women who smoked fewer than 10 cigarettes a day delivered children with a 25 percent higher chance of developing asthma than nonsmoking mothers.

In a 2006 study in *Respiratory Research,* investigators examined maternal smoking during pregnancy and the risk of recurring wheezing in infants during the first two years of life. The results show that any maternal smoking during pregnancy increases the risk of recurrent wheezing at age two. Infants were also at increased odds of being diagnosed with asthma if the mother smoked during pregnancy. Finally, exposure to secondhand smoke also increased the odds of recurrent wheezing and the diagnosis of asthma.

Q & A

Question: I've been smoking for several years now. After trying to quit a bunch of times, I've had no success. Is it just too late for me?

Answer: It's never too late to quit. Young people have an especially rough time trying to stop their smoking. Some need as many as 10 tries.

Look at each quitting attempt as practice. What went wrong that sent you back to smoking? How can you avoid that problem the next time around? Do you need more support from your friends and family? Maybe you need some professional help. Keep trying till you finish the job. For some, it's a case of "10th time lucky."

HOW TO GET SOME BREATHING ROOM

The first step in treating any respiratory condition is for the patient to stop smoking. It doesn't matter what the root cause of lung problems may be. Smoking aggravates the situation—as do fumes from other smokers.

See also: Body and Smoking, The; Cancer and Smoking; Secondhand Smoke

FURTHER READING

American Medical Association. *American Medical Association Family Medical Guide, 4th Edition.* Hoboken, N.J.: Wiley, 2004.

Goldmann, David R., ed. *American College of Physicians Complete Home Medical Guide.* New York: DK Publishing, 2003.

Ward, Jeremy P. T., Jane Ward, Richard M. Leach, and Charles M. Wiener. *The Respiratory System at a Glance.* Hoboken, N.J.: Wiley-Blackwell, 2005.

■ SECONDHAND SMOKE

Secondhand smoke, also known as **environmental tobacco smoke,** or ETS, is smoke from a cigarette that escapes into the air. When non-smokers breathe in these fumes, they are said to be engaged in passive smoking or involuntary smoking.

According to the Canadian Cancer Society, it takes approximately 12 minutes for an average cigarette to burn down. Smokers actually inhale for about 30 seconds during that 12-minute period. However, the output from a cigarette is roughly one-half mainstream smoke and one-half sidestream smoke. Mainstream smoke is drawn into the lungs of the smoker and breathed out again. Sidestream smoke comes from the lit tip of a cigarette.

Although the chemical properties of the two kinds of smoke are similar, they are not identical. When air isn't drawn through a cigarette, the tip is much cooler and the cigarette doesn't burn as efficiently, a condition known as incomplete combustion. As a result, sidestream smoke releases five times as much carbon monoxide and twice as much tar into the air compared to what enters a smoker's lungs. When chemists for R.J. Reynolds, a major tobacco company, investigated tobacco smoke, they found its pollution was 10,000 times more concentrated than auto exhausts on a highway during rush hour. Other chemists have discovered that the tar particles released in sidestream smoke, besides being more numerous, are only one-tenth the size of tar particles from mainstream smoke. Tinier size allows smoke particles to remain suspended in the air longer, leaving a haze and the distinctive smell of smoke in a room hours after a cigarette is finished. The concern, however, is about much more than a bad smell.

IS SECONDHAND SMOKE A CREDIBLE ISSUE?

In 1964, Surgeon General Luther L. Terry released a report linking smoking with cancer. Subsequent surgeons general released additional reports, including one in 1972 discussing "exposure to air pollution from tobacco smoke" and examining the dangers of smoking to the health of unborn children. As a result, several towns and cities began banning smoking in some public spaces.

The tobacco companies viewed the new laws as a threat. While Californians were voting on a referendum to restrict smoking in public buildings, the Tobacco Industry Research Committee, a public relations organization bankrolled by the tobacco companies, commissioned a poll by the Roper Organization.

The resulting report shrugged off several attacks made on the cigarette industry. The researchers warned, "The antismoking forces' latest tack, however—on the passive smoking issue—is quite a different matter . . . . Nearly six out of 10 believe that smoking is hazardous to the nonsmokers' health, up sharply over the last four years. More than two-thirds of nonsmokers believe it; nearly half of all smokers believe it."

The report goes on to explain, "What the smoker does to himself may be his business, but what the smoker does to the nonsmoker is quite a different matter. . . . This we see as the most dangerous development yet to the viability of the tobacco industry."

Tobacco companies responded to the report much as they had responded to news that smoking is linked to cancer many years earlier. They tried to convince the public that scientists disagreed about the effects of secondhand smoke. The goal was to keep people confused and doubtful about the issue. Cigarette companies funded supposedly independent foundations for research on indoor air quality and paid for articles and books to suggest a continuing controversy about secondhand smoke.

In 1992, the federal Environmental Protection Agency (EPA) prepared a major report on the risks of secondhand smoke. The EPA report stated that secondhand smoke caused cancers that kill 3,000 people a year. Fearing that the report would get wide circulation, cigarette companies attempted to kill it or delay its release using procedural tactics, lobbying in the White House, and even a lawsuit. Although the lawsuit failed in 2002, the cigarette manufacturers, led by the Philip Morris Corporation, had delayed and cast doubt on the report for 10 years.

Today, the Philip Morris web site has this to say on the subject: "Public health officials have concluded that secondhand smoke from cigarettes causes disease . . . . Philip Morris USA believes that the public should be guided by the conclusions of public health officials regarding the health effects of secondhand smoke in deciding whether to be in places where secondhand smoke is present, or if they are smokers, when and where to smoke around others."

TEENS SPEAK

Asthma and My Family's Smoking Habits

Chet is a tall, skinny high school freshman. He's never smoked.

"I can't remember not having asthma. When I was a little kid, I'd wheeze a lot. Sometimes I had trouble catching my breath.

"I guess the doctor caught it early. Whenever we went out, my mom always packed the inhaler along.

"Here's another thing. Both my parents smoked. It wasn't so bad with dad, because he was away at work, but mom would stay at home and smoke up a storm. It's an awful thing to say, but looking back, I had less bad days after I started going to school.

He shakes his head. "Dad quit smoking about five years ago. Mom kids him about it—he's gotten a little fatter since—but Mom, she can't quit. She's tried, but she ends up climbing the walls.

"When all this stuff about secondhand smoke began getting a lot of play on TV, I think Mom got sort of guilty. These days, when it's nice, she tries to take her smoke breaks out on our deck."

He starts coughing. "When she can't, I know about it the minute I get home."

Research has shown that secondhand smoke is a credible issue. The Centers for Disease Control estimates that between 22,700 and 69,600 premature deaths from heart disease can be attributed to secondhand smoke. The U.S. Environmental Protection Agency reports that secondhand smoke increases the risk of lower respiratory tract infections. The American Lung Association reports that approximately 3,400 lung cancer deaths each year can be attributed to secondhand smoke. Several other types of illnesses and deaths have been linked to secondhand smoke.

CHILDREN

The presence of secondhand smoke around children may have even more serious consequences than adults might face. Young children's bodies are still developing and may be more vulnerable to irritants in the environment. There are at least 40 dangerous chemicals among the 4,000 in cigarette smoke, so it is not surprising that children exposed to this smoke seem to get more illnesses.

In 1986, a pair of reports was issued on the connection between secondhand smoke and nonsmokers. Both the surgeon general's report and the report issued by the National Academy of Science's National Research Council found that secondhand smoke had negative effects on children. These findings were further confirmed by the EPA's 1992 report.

Children whose parents smoked had a higher rate of asthma, a medical condition where sudden swelling could choke off the air passages to the lungs. Medical researchers already knew that cigarette smoke triggered asthma attacks in adults. In children, they found evidence that smoke not only triggers more attacks, but more severe ones.

Children who breathe cigarette smoke consistently develop bronchial infections and pneumonia, coughs, wheezing, and ear infections. For very young children, secondhand smoke has been connected with sudden infant death syndrome (SIDS), a medical condition that occurs when a child under the age of one stops breathing, usually during the night, and suddenly dies without apparent cause.

Fact Or Fiction?

Smoking around other people won't hurt them.

The Facts: In 1604, King James I of England complained about secondhand smoke. As he put it, victims "must either take up smoking or resolve to live in a perpetual stinking torment."

Most nonsmokers probably feel the same way today, but they have more reasons to complain about smoking around them. As many as 73,000 people a year die from cancer and heart disease caused by breathing in other people's smoke.

In a 2005 study in *Environmental Health Perspectives*, researchers found that exposure to environmental tobacco smoke (ETS) hurt the cognitive abilities of children and adolescents. They measured exposure to ETS by examining serum cotinine levels in children and adolescents. Cotinine is a chemical that the body makes from nicotine. When a person is exposed to tobacco smoke, which contains nicotine, the body will start making cotinine. The more cotinine in the body, the more a person has been exposed to tobacco smoke.

The researchers found that as cotinine levels in the body increased, there was a decrease in reading, math, and visuospatial reasoning test scores. This means exposure to smoke hurts a child's ability to read, work out math problems, and use reasoning to solve problems.

SMOKING IN BUILDINGS

Moving air (wind or artificial ventilation) helps to move smoke away. However, hours after someone smoked in a room, visitors can still detect cigarette smoke. The reason is that the tiny particles from secondhand smoke do not go away quickly.

It's not easy to estimate the effects of secondhand smoke on a given workspace. The size of a room and its ventilation are straightforward, but other factors may vary. How many people will be smoking in the area? How many cigarettes will they smoke? In how much time? In most places where smoking is allowed, the "indoor pollution rate"—the amount of undispersed cigarette smoke in the air—remains too high. The solution suggested by many pro-smoking advocates—improved ventilation—is often expensive and may not solve the problem.

Cigarette smoke can irritate the eyes and cause allergic reactions, including asthma attacks. Irritants from smoke can also attack the nose, throat, the airways to the lungs, and the lungs themselves, resulting in blurred vision, wheezing, coughing, choking, and a considerable distraction from work in a workplace.

In an office environment, the odor is annoying, and the smoke is dirty. In a smoke-free office, drapes and upholstery require much less cleaning than in offices where smoking is allowed.

According to the Centers for Disease Control, by June 2008 there were 26 states with private sector workplace smoking bans. Twenty-five states banned smoking in restaurants, while 17 states banned smoking in bars.

The Centers for Disease Control state that by June 30, 2008, 26 states had implemented laws requiring private-sector worksites to be smoke-free. Twenty-one states required restaurants to be smoke-free. Only nine states had no smoking restrictions for restaurants. Seventeen states had implemented laws requiring bars to be smoke-free. In 2008, 28 states still had no smoking restrictions for bars.

The thorniest indoor smoking problem centers on the hospitality business—restaurants and bars. A large proportion of people who patronize these establishments—especially bars—are smokers. As a result, waiters, busboys, and bartenders work in an extremely smoky environment. However, attempts to make bars and restaurants smoke-free often results in angry letters from smoking patrons and complaints from owners that their business is being hurt. A major controversy over such regulations occurred in New York City when a smoking ban in restaurants and bars went into effect in 2003. One year later, antismoking activists hail the restrictions as a success, while opponents claim the ban has driven smokers from numerous bars and nightclubs, harming business while also damaging the city's reputation for nightlife.

Research on the economic impact of smoking bans has been positive. Contrary to the claims by the critics of these ordinances, bars and restaurants are not losing money because of smoke-free ordinances. One of the most well-known smoking bans occurred in New York City. Opponents of the ban predicted bars and restaurants would lose money and many would likely go out of business. An analysis of business tax receipts from restaurants and bars showed that the smoking ban did not hurt business. In fact, the tax receipts indicated an increase in business after the ban went into effect.

Results were similar in Florida. After a statewide smoking ban was enacted for restaurants, sales increased. Other data from around the United States shows the same trend. At a minimum, bars and restaurants do not lose money because of smoke-free ordinances.

Q & A

Question: My mom smokes a lot, even around my little sister. That worries me. Could it have something to do with the earaches my sister gets all the time?

Answer: Secondhand smoke around little kids can indeed cause an earache. It might be harder to talk about it with your mother than with a friend.

Look for items about secondhand smoke in the newspaper or TV news and call them to her attention. Or your might do a report on secondhand smoke for school and discuss it with her.

However you do it, have that conversation. Your mom and your sister may be grateful for it down the line.

WHAT REALLY ARE THE RISKS?

According to the CDC, about 3,400 nonsmokers die each year from lung cancer caused by breathing secondhand smoke.

As little as 20 minutes of exposure to secondhand smoke can make blood platelets "sticky," thickening the blood. This makes it harder for the heart to pump and raises the danger of blood clots, which can cause heart attack or stroke. According to the American Cancer Society, secondhand smoke causes between 35,000 and 40,000 deaths yearly among nonsmokers. Some research shows that women may be more susceptible to secondhand smoke.

Scientists have even designed physical tests to measure secondhand smoke exposure. They test breath for carbon monoxide and hair for nicotine. They've taken samples of saliva, blood, and urine to be checked for cotinine, a breakdown product of nicotine. These tests have shown the presence of secondhand smoke chemicals in the bodies of nonsmokers. Furthermore, some of these breakdown products came from cancer-causing compounds.

SOMETHING IN THE AIR

Since the first health questions about secondhand smoke were raised in the 1970s, the tobacco industry has tried to dismiss this problem as a mere annoyance, barely worth a cough. However, over three decades, evidence has mounted connecting cigarette smoke in the air with a number of illnesses suffered by nonsmokers. A vigorous effort by tobacco companies and various organizations funded by the tobacco industry has managed to confuse the issue but has not succeeded in disproving numerous studies showing problems such as asthma and respiratory problems in children and fatal consequences such as cancer and heart attack for adults can be traced

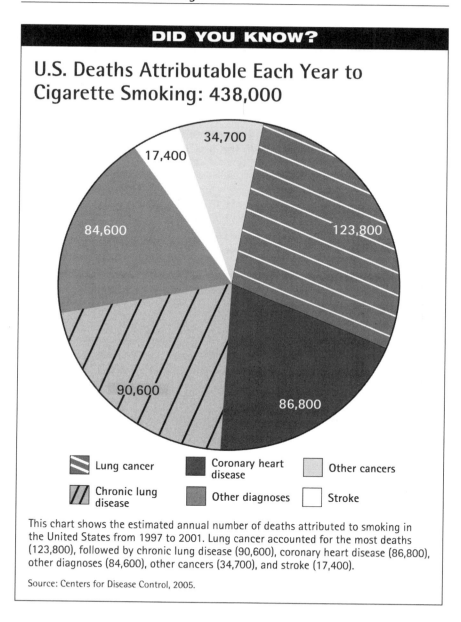

DID YOU KNOW?

U.S. Deaths Attributable Each Year to Cigarette Smoking: 438,000

34,700

17,400

84,600

123,800

90,600

86,800

☒ Lung cancer ■ Coronary heart disease ☐ Other cancers

▨ Chronic lung disease ▨ Other diagnoses ☐ Stroke

This chart shows the estimated annual number of deaths attributed to smoking in the United States from 1997 to 2001. Lung cancer accounted for the most deaths (123,800), followed by chronic lung disease (90,600), coronary heart disease (86,800), other diagnoses (84,600), other cancers (34,700), and stroke (17,400).

Source: Centers for Disease Control, 2005.

to secondhand smoke. Although cigarette industry delaying tactics have slowed the smoke-free workplace movement, smoking restrictions continue to be implemented across the country.

See also: Body and Smoking, The; Cardiovascular Disease and Smoking; Respiratory Diseases and Smoking

FURTHER READING

Glantz, Stanton A., John Slade, Lisa A. Bero, et al. *The Cigarette Papers.* Berkeley: University of California Press, 1996.

World Health Organization. *Protection from Exposure to Second-hand Tobacco Smoke: Policy Recommendations.* Geneva, Switzerland: World Health Organization, 2007.

■ SMOKING AND SOCIETY

In American society since colonial times, tobacco has played an important role. In Virginia and other southern colonies, tobacco was the main cash crop. In the early years of the United States, many men and some women smoked tobacco in pipes and cigars. In the 1880s, cigarettes began to be mass-produced and became an important consumer item. For the first half of the 20th century, cigarette sales rose steeply, and the cigarette became entrenched in the social life of the United States.

In 1964, Surgeon General Luther L. Terry, the government's highest health official, issued the first report linking cigarette smoking with cancer and other diseases. At the time this report came out, cigarette ads ran on television every day, and every office had an ashtray. Smoking was very much a part of life, and smokers seemed to be a majority—as numerous as the cigarettes that marched endlessly in ads across the nation's TV screens.

American female smokers were a minority. While 51.9 percent of men smoked, only 33.9 percent of women were smokers. As more information on the dangers of smoking continued to come out, the percentage of smokers shrank to 20.8 percent of the population by 2008.

CALIFORNIA SETS THE STANDARD
FOR ANTISMOKING TRENDS

California often sets trends for the rest for the country. Certainly, that has been true when it comes to smoking. The first city in the United States to restrict smoking in some public places was Berkeley, California, in 1977. California voters considered several statewide attempts to establish smoking limitations in following years, but these referendums failed to pass.

In 1980, San Luis Obispo became the first city in the world to ban smoking in all public buildings, including bars and restaurants. The University of California in San Francisco struck a major blow against the tobacco companies in 1994 when an unknown individual leaked thousands of pages of secret documents from Brown & Williamson, a major tobacco corporation, to a professor at the school. Through the university's library, these "cigarette papers" were opened to the public. When Brown & Williamson sued to prevent this, the California Supreme Court rejected the claim. The papers contained all sorts of damaging information that was made available on the Internet. In 1998, California became the first state to ban smoking in bars, continuing the battle on secondhand smoke.

Adopted in 1988, California's five-point program for tobacco control became a model for the rest of the nation:

- Increase the prices of tobacco products through higher taxes

- Use community-based programs to educate the public on the dangers of smoking

- Establish smoke-free workplaces and public spaces

- Support programs to help people quit smoking

- Run counteradvertising campaigns to remove the appeal of smoking

After 11 years of these policies (1988 through 1999) California enjoyed the second-lowest smoking rate in the country, as well as steep reductions in cancer rates. (The state with the lowest smoking rate is Utah, due to the large Mormon population. The Church of Jesus Christ of Latter-Day Saints disapproves of smoking.)

The California Department of Public Health found that between 2004 and 2006, smoking rates for young people increased. In 2004, 13.2 percent of high school youth reported smoking in the last 30 days. By 2006, this figure was up to 15.4 percent. That is still below the national average of 19.7 percent.

SOCIAL IMPACT FOR ADULTS

Since the surgeon general's report in 1964, attitudes about smoking and smokers have changed in small and large ways. In the 1970s, nonsmokers formed groups to protect their rights and raise questions about the health dangers of secondhand smoke, the tobacco smoke left in the air by burning cigarettes and breathed in by everyone nearby. By the 1980s, as more localities began establishing smoking restrictions, smokers found fewer places to indulge in their habit. In 1990, Congress banned smoking on all U.S. domestic flights. By 1999, smoking was also banned on international flights. That year, 79 percent of workplaces with at least 50 or more employees banned smoking or limited it to special areas. Restaurants advertised smoke-free areas, and in some communities, local governments voted to keep all public places smoke-free.

Secondhand smoke was no longer only a problem just for non-smokers. Now it was a problem for the people who smoked. In the 1960s, the phrase "Mind if I smoke?" was less a courtesy than an announcement: "I'm going to smoke." By the end of the 20th century, more and more nonsmokers *did* mind. A draft report for the federal Environmental Protection Agency noted that 46 percent of respondents to an opinion poll expressed annoyance with secondhand smoke in 1964. By 1987, 69 percent objected to it.

Among the many secret tobacco documents made public by leaks or through court cases was a 1982 survey of smokers commissioned by R.J. Reynolds, a major cigarette manufacturer. According to the survey, 60 percent of the respondents faced restrictions on smoking at work. The most surprising answer on the survey, however, dealt with smoking restrictions in public spaces like restaurants and bars. An overwhelming majority—79 percent—of smokers who had to live with these restrictions *approved* of them.

The report explained the discrepancy by saying that smokers were becoming increasingly unsure about how welcome their habit would be. Restrictions, in a way, became reassuring. There were still places that could be considered safe territory.

Q & A

Question: I help out at my grandfather's store after school until my folks get off from work. Granddad is pretty cool for an old guy. He leaves his pack of cigarettes on his office desk and says, "I used to grab a smoke whenever I could when I was a kid. I guess kids today aren't any different." Should I take him up on his offer?

Answer: When your grandfather was young, teen smoking was considered "just something kids do." Your grandfather began smoking back then and apparently has been smoking ever since. As an adult, that's his choice.

The question is, do you want to make what may be a lifelong commitment to be a smoker, even if a "cool person" invites you? Much more evidence has piled up on the dangers of smoking since your grandfather's youth. You may want to consider the evidence before you make a life choice that can be very hard to undo.

SOCIAL IMPACT FOR TEENS

Attitudes about teen smoking have also changed in the last 40 years. What was once considered a minor vice has become a major problem. Since the 1980s, tobacco companies have been criticized for aiming advertising at young people, even grade-school students. Efforts to reduce the number of young smokers have met with varying results. The 1990s saw an upswing in smoking among youth, due in part, many believed, to the Joe Camel ad campaign. A cartoon character with an edgy image, Joe made smoking look glamorous to a lot of young people. In recent years, youth smoking has dropped, except for a surprising new development. In the 2002 National Survey on Drug Use and Health (NSDUH), cigarette use in the youngest age group (12–17 years) showed more female than male smokers. Since 2002, teen smoking has continued to drop. More females than males continue to smoke, although the difference is not significant.

For teen smokers today, the reality of smoking is very different from the confident, cool images shown in the media. According to the 2006 National Survey on Drug Use and Health, cigarette use is highest among those who never finished high school (35.6 percent) and those who are unemployed (47.8 percent).

In a 2007 report by Columbia University's Center on Addiction and Substance Abuse (CASA), researchers found that smoking is a good predictor of drug use. The study focused on teenagers who were 12 to 17 years old. According to the report, teens who smoke are more than 8.5 times as likely to use illicit drugs as nonsmoking teens. More than 63 percent of teenage marijuana smokers also smoke cigarettes, and almost 45 percent who use other illicit drugs also smoke cigarettes.

SOCIETAL COSTS

As social attitudes toward smoking changed, many smokers became aware of the personal costs associated with their habit. Depending on the severity of their health problems, some lost their teeth, their ability to work, or even their lives. Beyond the personal losses are other costs connected to smoking.

Could consumers trust the safety of the products they buy? Should state governments demand additional payments from companies that make legal products and pay heavy taxes on them? Should employers and insurance companies discriminate against people because of their lifestyle choices?

LAWSUITS

In 1952, *Reader's Digest* published an article entitled "Cancer by the Carton," the first article to inform a national audience about the connection between smoking and cancer. Within two years, cancer patients began suing tobacco companies to recover the costs of their medical care. Lawyers argued that cigarette companies failed to warn customers about the cancer dangers in their product. Therefore they should be held liable for damages. For decades, tobacco companies won these cases.

In 1994, the most serious attempt to sue tobacco companies took shape as 60 law firms from across the country joined forces to file a class action in federal court. A class action covers all those who have been harmed by an action. The lawsuit demanded that the tobacco companies pay damages not for getting people sick, but for lying to them about the addictive power of nicotine.

Then in 1996, a federal appeals court struck down the case. Judges found that the circumstances of the 90 million individuals involved were too different and that the state laws involved in the case were also too dissimilar. The judges also commented on the unprecedented size of the case and the threat it presented—a single jury deciding the fate of millions of people and a major industry. The law firms then launched class-action suits in all fifty states. Although many of these cases were also thrown out of court, in 2003, a Florida jury awarded the smokers $145 million in punitive damages, the largest amount ever awarded in a civil lawsuit. This decision was later reversed on appeal.

The cigarette companies had averted one major threat, but they faced an even more serious challenge. In 1995, Michael Moore, Mississippi's attorney general (the head lawyer for the state), filed a lawsuit against the tobacco companies to recover the money that the state spent

DID YOU KNOW?

State Tobacco-Related Costs and Revenues, 2006

(all amounts in millions of dollars except where otherwise indicated)

State	Smoking-Caused Health Costs	Smoking-Caused Productivity Losses	State Gov't Smoking Medicaid Costs	Federal Smoking-Caused Costs	Other State Government Smoking Health Costs	Other Fed. Smoking Caused Costs	Taxpayers Fed/State Tax Burden From
States Total	$96+ bill.	$97+ bill.	$13.3 bill.	$17.6 bill.	$2.9+ bill.	$37 bill.	$70+ bill.
Alabama	$1.49 bill.	$2.05 bill.	$74.1	$163.8	$45.0	$588.3	$986.8
Alaska	$169	$157	$37.6	$39.3	$5.1	$77.7	$155.8
Arizona	$1.3 bill.	$1.49 bill	$105.9	$210.0	$38.6	$725.2	$1.2 bill.
Arkansas	$812	$1.3 bill.	$64.4	$177.5	$24.4	$358.9	$616.3
California	$9.14 bill.	$8.58 bill.	$1.47 bill.	$1.47 bill.	$274.3	$4.0 bill.	$7.6 bill.
Colorado	$1.31 bill.	$992	$159.5	$159.5	$39.4	$599.4	$1.0 bill.
Connecticut	$1.63 bill.	$1.01 bill.	$215.0	$215.0	$48.9	$436.6	$906.1
Delaware	$284	$304	$39.5	$39.5	$8.5	$103.6	$202.1
DC	$243	$233	$23.4	$54.6	$7.3	$81.4	$151.1
Florida	$6.32 bill.	$6.47 bill.	$515.5	$734.5	$189.6	$2.3 bill.	$4.1 bill.
Georgia	$2.25 bill.	$3.08 bill.	$204.2	$332.7	$67.6	$1.1 bill.	$1.8 bill.

State	State Smoking-Caused Health Costs	Smoking-Caused Productivity Losses	Other Gov't Smoking Medicaid Costs	Other Federal Smoking-Caused Costs	Taxpayers State Government Smoking Health Costs	Other Fed. Smoking Caused Costs	Taxpayers Fed/State Tax Burden From
States Total	$96+ bill.	$97+ bill.	$13.3 bill.	$17.6 bill.	$2.9+ bill.	$37 bill.	$70+ bill.
Hawaii	$336	$308	$49.6	$67.3	$10.1	$140.6	$268.3
Idaho	$319	$332	$24.6	$58.3	$9.6	$173.9	$292.3
Illinois	$4.10 bill.	$4.29 bill.	$785.0	$785.0	$123.2	$1.5 bill.	$3.1 bill.
Indiana	$2.08 bill.	$2.49 bill.	$182.0	$304.9	$62.5	$802.9	$1.4 bill.
Iowa	$1.01 bill	$964	$114.4	$186.5	$30.5	$395.9	$727.4
Kansas	$927	$863	$77.9	$118.0	$27.8	$351.5	$625.7
Kentucky	$1.50 bill.	$2.13 bill.	$148.1	$338.8	$45.0	$543.9	$995.4
Louisiana	$1.47 bill.	$1.91 bill.	$200.9	$462.0	$44.2	$551.3	$1,058.5
Maine	$602	$495	$79.3	$136.6	$18.1	$177.6	$360.4
Maryland	$1.96 bill.	$1.78 bill.	$238.0	$238.0	$58.9	$688.2	$1.3 bill.
Massachusetts	$3.54 bill.	$1.92 bill.	$523.0	$523.0	$106.3	$806.6	$1.8 bill.
Michigan	$3.40 bill.	$3.8 bill.	$492.0	$635.9	$102.0	$1.3 bill.	$2.4 bill.
Minnesota	$2.06 bill.	$1.2 bill.	$232.5	$232.5	$61.9	$666.0	$1.2 bill.
Mississippi	$719	$1.41 bill.	$63.6	$200.3	$21.6	$355.2	$611.0
Missouri	$2.13 bill.	$2.41 bill.	$204.2	$327.7	$64.1	$751.1	$1.3 bill.
Montana	$277	$294	$20.6	$46.3	$8.3	$122.1	$207.6
Nebraska	$537	$499	$56.3	$77.6	$16.1	$229.4	$409.9

(continues)

State Tobacco-Related Costs and Revenues, 2006 (continued)

State	State Smoking-Caused Health Costs	Smoking-Caused Productivity Losses	Other Gov't Smoking Medicaid Costs	Other Federal Smoking-Caused Costs	Taxpayers State Government Smoking Health Costs	Other Fed. Smoking Caused Costs	Taxpayers Fed/State Tax Burden From
States Total	$96+ bill.	$97+ bill.	$13.3 bill.	$17.6 bill.	$2.9+ bill.	$37 bill.	$70+ bill.
Nevada	$565	$832	$56.6	$66.3	$17.0	$299.7	$513.4
New Hampshire	$564	$405	$57.5	$57.5	$16.9	$162.8	$315.5
New Jersey	$3.17 bill.	$2.62 bill.	$483.5	$483.5	$95.3	$1.0 bill.	$2.1 bill.
New Mexico	$461	$467	$51.6	$132.3	$13.8	$240.5	$418.5
New York	$8.17 bill.	$6.01 bill.	$2.73 bill.	$2.73 bill.	$245.1	$2.3 bill.	$6.4 bill.
North Carolina	$2.46 bill.	$3.3 bill.	$272.8	$496.1	$73.9	$1.1 bill.	$2.0 bill.
North Dakota	$247	$190	$16.5	$30.4	$7.4	$88.8	$155.1
Ohio	$4.37 bill.	$4.65 bill.	$575.2	$850.7	$131.3	$1.5 bill.	$2.8 bill.
Oklahoma	$1.16 bill.	$1.55 bill.	$69.4	$148.5	$34.9	$455.1	$774.0
Oregon	$1.11 bill.	$1.07 bill.	$111.7	$175.2	$33.5	$469.9	$836.6
Pennsylvania	$5.19 bill.	$4.63 bill.	$779.9	$930.0	$155.8	$1.6 bill.	$3.2 bill.
Rhode Island	$506	$364	$85.2	$93.7	$15.2	$133.2	$297.4
South Carolina	$1.09 bill.	$1.83 bill.	$119.7	$273.2	$32.9	$540.2	$946.1
South Dakota	$274	$228	$21.5	$36.4	$8.2	$103.6	$180.2
Tennessee	$2.16 bill.	$2.74 bill.	$247.1	$432.8	$65.0	$780.7	$1.4 bill.

State	State Smoking-Caused Health Costs	Smoking-Caused Productivity Losses	Other Gov't Smoking Medicaid Costs	Other Federal Smoking-Caused Costs	Taxpayers State Government Smoking Health Costs	Other Fed. Smoking Caused Costs	Taxpayers Fed/State Tax Burden From
States Total	$96+ bill.	$97+ bill.	$13.3 bill.	$17.6 bill.	$2.9+ bill.	$37 bill.	$70+ bill.
Texas	$5.83 bill.	$6.44 bill.	$635.3	$984.6	$174.9	$2.6 bill.	$4.6 bill.
Utah	$345	$274	$31.0	$72.9	$10.4	$259.0	$425.5
Vermont	$233	$197	$29.5	$42.4	$7.0	$81.4	$157.2
Virginia	$2.08 bill.	$2.42 bill.	$200.5	$200.5	$62.6	$950.9	$1.6 bill.
Washington	$1.95 bill.	$1.74 bill.	$324.7	$326.2	$58.7	$806.6	$1.5 bill.
West Virginia	$690	$994	$62.2	$166.7	$20.7	$244.2	$442.2
Wisconsin	$2.02 bill.	$1.64 bill.	$204.1	$275.8	$60.7	$732.6	$1.3 bill.
Wyoming	$136	$155	$17.4	$19.5	$4.1	$66.6	$120.9

Tobacco-related costs are in the billions of dollars. Smoking-related health costs are more than $96 billion. Also, more than $70 billion in taxes went to the state and federal governments to help cover smoking-related costs (such as Medicaid).

Source: Campaign for Tobacco-Free Kids.

treating people for tobacco-related illnesses. He started a trend that ended with similar suits from all 50 states. Four states—Texas, Florida, Mississippi, and Minnesota—settled separately. After years of negotiations, the remaining state lawsuits were also settled out of court.

Under the terms of what became known as the Master Settlement Agreement (MSA) signed in 1998, the tobacco companies agreed to pay the states $205 billion over 25 years. The agreement also set aside $1.7 billion to create the American Legacy Foundation, an organization to educate the public and help protect young people from tobacco products.

As part of the agreement, tobacco companies also agreed to dissolve several organizations they had funded to promote smoking and counteract criticism of the industry. The companies also agreed to stop advertising to young people and on billboards. Many corporate papers which had been secret were now opened to the public.

Antitobacco activists complained that the MSA didn't go far enough. It didn't punish the cigarette manufacturers. They were allowed to go on with their business and pass the heavy costs of the settlement onto the shoulders of cigarette smokers through higher prices.

However thanks to the settlement, the American Legacy Foundation was able to launch its "Truth" campaign, the first major nationwide advertising campaign against cigarettes in 30 years. Price hikes on cigarettes also contributed to a downturn in smoking.

Fact Or Fiction?

That big tobacco settlement is really going to cost the cigarette companies.

The Facts: Actually, the settlement will cost cigarette smokers. Between 1998 and 2006, tobacco companies raised the price of cigarettes by about $1.25 a pack. Not only are smokers paying off the settlement, they're creating large new profits for the tobacco companies.

COST OF HEALTH COVERAGE

In recent decades, health-care costs have risen, and so has the cost of insurance. Companies have begun asking employees to pay for some of this cost. This has led to a new controversy over smoking.

Group health plans are a way to get coverage at a "wholesale price" by spreading the risk. Payments for single employees help bring down the cost of health care for workers with many children. Healthy young workers with little need for doctors help to cover the costs for older employees.

Forced to reach into their own pockets, however, employees have started looking at health care in a new light. Is it fair for everyone to pay for people who are more likely to get sick—especially if they bring it on themselves with lifestyle choices like overeating or smoking? Should health coverage be like some life insurance policies, where nonsmokers get to pay less?

A 2006 survey by a health insurance company found that 60 percent of respondents believed a person's lifestyle choices should affect how much that person pays for health insurance. Sixty-six percent felt that smokers should pay higher premiums than nonsmokers. By comparison, 37 percent felt someone who is obese should pay higher premiums than someone who is not obese.

PREMATURE DEATH AND DISABILITY

On average, male smokers live 13.2 years less than nonsmokers. Female smokers lose 14.5 years off their expected life spans. When you add up the number of people who die from smoking-related causes, that cost gets very high. According to a 2005 report from the Centers for Disease Control and Prevention (CDC), productivity losses in the United States from smokers' deaths averaged almost $92 billion per year between 1997 and 2001.

The CDC reports that in 1998, $75.5 billion was spent on smoking-attributable health-care expenses. From 1997 through 2001, health-care expenditures and productivity losses were more than $167 billion per year.

The Centers for Medicare & Medicaid Services (CMMS), the government agency which tracks health-care programs, reported that Americans spent $2.1 trillion on health care in 2006. Private spending was $1.1 trillion. **Medicare**, the federal health-care benefits program for the elderly and permanently disabled, cost taxpayers $401 billion. **Medicaid**, a health insurance program for those with low income that has its costs shared by federal and state governments, came in at $309 billion. According to a Columbia University study of 1995 health costs, 14 percent of Medicare spending went to treating tobacco-related diseases. The diseases also accounted for 6.6 percent of Medicaid costs in 1996, according to a study for the Robert Wood Johnson Foundation. If these percentages are applied to the 2006 numbers, they give some idea of the large sums of money involved. According to the CMMS, one study estimates that Medicare spends 10 percent of its annual budget on treating smoking-related illnesses.

YOUR STATE DOLLARS AT WORK

In 2006, the Organization for Tobacco-Free Kids, an antismoking action group, found that tobacco-related Medicaid costs for all 50 states totaled more than $13.3 billion. The states also faced an additional $2.9 billion for smoking-related problems.

States with large populations and generous Medicaid benefits faced steep expenses. California paid $1.47 billion. New York faced a bill of more than $2.7 billion. Most states ranged from $20 million to hundreds of millions of dollars for the year.

Although yearly payments from the Master Settlement Agreement with the tobacco companies were supposed to cover these costs, cash-strapped states like New Jersey and Washington are often using that money to cover budget deficits. Some have even securitized their settlement monies, essentially taking out a loan on their promised payments for a one-time cash amount.

To protect their settlement payments, state governments have even stepped into other tobacco lawsuits on the tobacco companies' side. In 2003, when a judge imposed a $12 billion bond on the Philip Morris Company, 37 states joined the tobacco company to have the bond reduced. Their reason? Heavy judgments on tobacco companies might drive them into bankruptcy and stop the MSA payments.

See also: Government and Tobacco; Smoking, History of; Cost of Smoking

FURTHER READING

Gately, Iain. *Tobacco.* New York: Grove Press, 2002.
Goel, Rajeev K., and Michael A. Nelson. *Global Efforts to Conbat Smoking.* Burlington, Vt.: Ashgate, 2008.

■ SMOKING, HISTORY OF

The long history of tobacco use, first in the Western Hemisphere, and in more recent centuries, in countries around the world.

THE BEGINNINGS

The tobacco plant is native to the Americas. For more than 2,000 years, native peoples in both North America and South America used tobacco as a medicine and in religious observances. The ancient Mayan civilization in Mexico considered tobacco to be a kind of incense and burned it to ask the gods for rain during droughts. As part of their religious ceremonies, Mayans also smoked a very strong variety of tobacco that caused hallucinations. The earliest representation of smoking occurs on a piece of Mayan pottery found in Guatemala. The decoration, showing a man smoking a cigar, was made more than 1,000 years ago.

When Christopher Columbus first set foot in the Western Hemisphere in 1492, Native Americans gave him gifts—fruits and strong-smelling leaves. Columbus served the fruit to his sailors, but threw the leaves—tobacco—overboard.

In time, however, Spanish and other visitors to the Americas learned to smoke the tobacco leaves. Within 200 years, European sailors had spread the habit around the world. In Korea, for instance, smoking was well established by 1620—about 10 years before it reached Sweden.

Smoking was not always welcomed. At various times, the practice was denounced by the pope in Italy, made a criminal act in Turkey and most of the Middle East, and could result in exile to Siberia in Russia.

Native Americans not only smoked tobacco in cigars and pipes but also in cigarettes, according to Spanish explorers in Mexico. European cigarette smoking began in the Spanish city of Seville, where beggars disassembled cigar butts and wrapped the tobacco in scraps of paper.

In 1560, Jean Nicot, the French ambassador to Portugal, sent reports on tobacco and plants to the royal court. When tobacco was first introduced to Europe, it was considered a medicinal herb, the same status it had in the Americas. Throughout the 1500s and 1600s, doctors used tobacco to cure or relieve numerous diseases, including cancer.

In the 1560s, English sailors also brought tobacco back to their homeland. Although the credit is given to Captain John Hawkins, other English seafarers may have introduced the plant to the English even earlier.

In 1606 King James I of England wrote a book called *A Counterblaste to Tobacco,* a scathing attack on smoking. James also raised the tax on tobacco 4,000 percent. During this time, tobacco was very expensive because it was imported from Spain. However, when tobacco began to be shipped from Virginia in 1614, the king lowered the tax and made the trade a royal monopoly. Apparently, economics overcame the king's dislike of smoking.

Tobacco was the first profitable crop for the struggling English colony in Virginia. Instead of cultivating the rough-tasting local tobacco, colonist John Rolfe imported plants from islands in the Caribbean Sea. Rolfe sent this better-tasting tobacco to England in 1612. It became popular, and a thriving trade developed. Within seven years, tobacco became the leading cash crop for Virginia. Eventually, tobacco became the economic basis for all of England's southern colonies.

Cultivation of tobacco required considerable work and many workers. In early Virginia, this labor was first performed by indentured servants, individuals who traded several years of service for passage to the new colony, or by captured Native Americans. In 1619, a Dutch ship visiting Virginia traded a group of Africans for supplies. At first these newcomers were regarded as indentured servants, but as more Africans arrived, they were enslaved. By that time, African slaves soon became an important part of the colonial economy.

When the North American colonists finally declared themselves independent of Britain in 1776, tobacco played a part in the struggle. The export helped the colonists secure loans in Europe to bring weapons and supplies for George Washington's army.

For years during the early days of the United States, tobacco was the new nation's number one export. In fact, tobacco was the primary American export until the early 1800s, when cotton took over.

Tobacco affected not only the economy of the new United States but also the country's culture. People saw tobacco as a symbol, a distinctly American crop sold all over the world. This pride turns up in an architectural detail in the nation's capital. Washington's domed Capitol building, the home of the U.S. Congress, features a set of columns erected in the 1840s. The tops of these pillars depict corn (another American crop) and tobacco plants.

Agricultural products such as tobacco and cotton brought wealth to the southern states, but that wealth was based on slavery. Many in the North began to speak out against the practice of owning slaves, and the country divided in a bitter argument. In 1861, 11 southern states seceded from the Union, starting a civil war.

The Civil War (1861–1865) introduced soldiers to a new kind of tobacco—gold leaf. The variety is also known as "bright leaf" tobacco because its leaves turn a bright golden color when dried over charcoal fires. Farmers in upper North Carolina and lower Virginia were just beginning to develop a market for gold leaf when the war began.

During the war, soldiers from both sides developed a taste for the new tobacco. Their interest led to the rise of the first major tobacco brand in the United States, Bull Durham.

CIGARETTES: AN AMERICAN SUCCESS STORY

The century after the Civil War was a time of great success for the tobacco industry. During those years, cigarette manufacturing changed from a handmade process to one that relied on machines.

Cigarette manufacturing required many workers, since the product had to be rolled by hand. In the 1860s, many tobacco companies imported skilled cigarette rollers from Europe. In 1881, the Duke family brought 125 Russian immigrants to Durham, North Carolina, to roll cigarettes and teach the task to others. Many local women became cigarette rollers.

In 1883, the Duke family gambled by purchasing the first cigarette-making machine. By 1884, the Dukes were rolling out 744 million cigarettes annually, more than all of the cigarette companies in the nation had made the previous year.

The new machine lowered the cost of producing cigarettes, and the transcontinental railroads opened new markets. Color printing spurred the growth of advertising, which the Dukes used to create a market for the flood of cigarettes from their factories. By 1904, the Dukes' American Tobacco Company held a **monopoly** over the cigarette business in the United States, controlling both prices and production.

In 1900, only 5 percent of the U.S. population smoked cigarettes. Chewing tobacco was much more popular. Few could imagine the future success of cigarettes, least of all a British company which set up a U.S. operation to import its products in 1902. The company was Philip Morris.

The early decades of the 20th century were marked by a distrust of monopolies. In 1911, the federal government broke up the American Tobacco Company through an antitrust suit. The giant corporation was broken into several companies that immediately began competing to see who could get the largest share of the market. R.J. Reynolds scored the greatest success, launching its Camel brand with a new mix of cigarette tobaccos and a brilliant advertising campaign. By the time the United States entered World War I in 1917, Camels had cornered one-third of the American cigarette market.

Military service introduced millions of young men to cigarettes, which were packaged as part of their rations. By the end of World War I in 1918, many of the returning soldiers were confirmed smokers. By

1924, American tobacco users were evenly divided between cigarette smokers and tobacco chewers.

The 1930s continued to see more and more smokers in the United States as smoking by women became more accepted. Tobacco companies sponsored many of the most popular shows on radio, the new entertainment medium.

The United States entered World War II in 1941, and again, American soldiers and sailors went to war with cigarettes as part of their rations. Servicemen returned home as confirmed smokers and pushed the percentage of American smokers even higher.

Smoking levels continued to rise through the 1950s as cigarette companies began advertising on yet another new medium, television. By the 1960s the United States had more smokers than ever before. In 1964, 51.9 percent of American males and 33.9 percent of American females smoked cigarettes.

Beginning in 1962, the head of the federal government's public health service, Surgeon General Luther L. Terry, assembled a group of scientists and medical professionals to examine the available research on the health effects of cigarette smoking. Some believe the project had been commissioned by then president John F. Kennedy. Dr. Terry was himself a smoker until he began working on the report. Issued in 1964, the document that came to be known as the surgeon general's report made a connection between smoking and three diseases: lung cancer, cancer of the larynx (voicebox), and chronic bronchitis (inflammation of the air passages leading to the lungs).

GROWING DIFFICULTIES

The report did not contain new findings. As early as the 1930s, researchers had been finding links between cigarette smoking and a variety of illnesses, but studies were rarely publicized.

The 1960s and 1970s were confusing times for smokers. Tobacco companies fought the news of health risks associated with smoking, launching a public relations counterattack that has come to be known as the "smokescreen." Nonetheless, the percentage of smokers began to decline. In 1971, cigarette commercials were banned from television and radio, another blow for the tobacco industry.

In the same period, however, some cigarette brands enjoyed unprecedented success. Philip Morris created a new tobacco formula for Marlboros and an advertising campaign that made the "Marlboro Man" an international sales icon. Marlboro had not even placed among the top 10 cigarette sellers in 1950. By 1972, the brand had become the top-selling cigarettes in the world.

The 1980s saw a growth of restrictions on smokers as localities and states enacted regulations for smoking in government buildings, schools, workplaces, restaurants, and bars, a process which goes on to the present day. In 1987, the Joe Camel advertising campaign was launched. Youth smoking, which had been declining, proceeded to go up the following year.

Tobacco companies managed to defeat regulation attempts both by Congress and the Food and Drug Administration regarding advertising, new health warnings on cigarette packs, and making most public places smoke-free. In the courts, however, they faced serious legal challenges as the attorneys general of all 50 states sued to recover health-care costs for people with tobacco-related illnesses. The cases were finally settled out of court in 1998 with the signing of the Master Settlement Agreement. The tobacco companies agreed to pay the states $206 billion over 25 years and received new restrictions on advertising and promotion, especially to young people.

Less than one-quarter of the population smokes today. Though on the defensive, tobacco companies retain considerable political, economic, and legal power.

TOBACCO AND WORLD AFFAIRS

As the U.S. market for cigarettes continued to grow smaller, tobacco companies were left with excess manufacturing capacity. The result—the tobacco industry began aggressively marketing to the rest of the world.

Tobacco companies have always been international firms, marketing their brands in many countries. For the last two decades, however, the industry has focused its marketing on developing nations. Although these efforts may bring in new profits for the tobacco corporations, they also bring new health problems to countries in need of doctors and hospitals.

The economic stakes are high. More than 5.5 trillion cigarettes are produced worldwide—per day. Over 350 million people smoke in China alone. American cigarette makers want a share of that market. Since the 1980s, the U.S. government has helped, putting pressure on countries like Japan, Thailand, and South Korea to open their markets to American cigarettes.

Exports reached a high point in 1996, when American companies shipped 243 billion cigarettes to foreign markets. That number dropped to 109.9 billion in 2006, but the export trade still brought in $1.2 billion. The United States is even exporting its famous gold leaf tobacco, not just processed leaves, but the plants themselves. American companies have encouraged farmers around to world to start growing bright leaf tobacco. The idea is to give countries that grow harsher strains of the plant a taste of American tobacco—and, hopefully, a taste for American cigarettes.

Today one-half of the tobacco in American cigarettes comes from foreign countries, undercutting prices for American tobacco and driving many small farmers out of business. By heavily mechanizing and opening new tobacco plants overseas, transnational tobacco corporations are exporting manufacturing jobs to developing countries as well.

TEENS SPEAK

A Dying Tradition?

Roy is a big, soft-spoken 21-year-old. Since graduating high school he's kept up two part-time jobs while also working on his family's farm. He's smoked since he was 15.

"I would be—should be—the fifth generation of my family to work this farm." He brushes sweat off his forehead with the back of his hand. "It's not a big place, but we were always able to keep our heads above water by keeping a few acres in tobacco. Thing was, a farmer could get $4,000 an acre. That could make all the difference in a lean year.

"Even with what I made coming in, my Daddy spent a lot of his time off the farm, doing other jobs to keep us going. In fact, he was miles from here when he just sort of fell over. Heart attack. He shouldn't have gone so young, but they say it was because of his smoking.

Roy shrugs. "We all smoke in this family—always did. But with Daddy gone, that leaves me to carry on. I don't know if I can do it. The tobacco isn't making the same kind of money, and there's nothing else I can plant in those couple of acres to make the same kind of profit. We can hang on for this year, but next year? Our family farm may just be a part of someone else's operation."

TOBACCO TODAY IN THE UNITED STATES

The most recent figures, from 2006, offer a snapshot on the status of smoking in the United States. That year, smokers consumed 371 billion cigarettes.

In 2006, approximately 45.3 million Americans (age 18 and older) smoked, about 21 percent of the population. The group with the largest percentage of smokers was the youngest, 18–24 years old. The lowest percentage could be found among those over 65.

Statistics for 2006 show that American smokers consumed fewer cigarettes than they used to. In 1974, only 31.6 percent smoked fewer than 15 cigarettes a day. By 2006, 53 percent smoked fewer than 15 cigarettes daily. In the same time period, the group smoking 15–24 cigarettes a day group shrank from 43.2 percent to 34.9 percent. Those who smoked over 24 cigarettes a day were down by 50 percent. The surgeon general's report of 1989 suggests that the decline may be due in part to people having fewer places to smoke and therefore fewer opportunities do so. By 2004, every state had some sort of restriction on indoor smoking. Some states set aside certain areas where smoking is allowed. Others ban or limit smoking in almost all public places. Some 46 states restricted smoking in government workplaces, and 25 have extended those limits to private workplaces as well.

Educational differences in tobacco use

According to the American Lung Association, in 2006, about 26.8 percent of adults without a high school diploma were smokers. For those who graduated college, only 8.8 percent were smokers.

Fact Or Fiction?

You may not like Big Tobacco, but at least they're American companies.

The Facts: Actually, the largest tobacco companies are transnational corporations, with operations in many countries. In recent years, they've been moving both farming and manufacturing operations overseas. The American market still provides tremendous profits. But the largest companies, like Philip Morris and R.J. Reynolds, seem to be keeping their options open if American profits fall too far down or American regulation rises too high.

Regional tobacco use

Kentucky, with its history as a tobacco-producing state, has the highest percentage of smokers. It also has one of the lowest taxes on tobacco in the country. Nevada, the next highest state for smoking, owes its position to gambling. State law allows smoking wherever gambling occurs. Since slot machines can be found almost anywhere—including supermarkets and laundromats—people are free to smoke in areas where smoking would be banned in other states.

Utah's status as the state with the lowest percentage of smokers is due to its large population of Mormons, whose religion strongly disapproves of the habit. California's place as the second-lowest smoking state (only 14.9 percent of Californians are smokers) results from decades of tobacco control and smoking education. In 1977, the city of Berkeley passed the first law to limit smoking in restaurants and public places. Statewide smoking restrictions were discussed in a 1978 referendum which was defeated.

In 1998, however, Proposition 10, imposing a 50 cents per pack tax on cigarettes, passed after an extremely close vote. Many Hollywood celebrities campaigned for the tax, which would fund tobacco education and social services. With more than seven million votes cast, 50.4 percent of Californians supported the initiative.

Q & A

Question: I'm really stressing out at school and at home. My friend keeps offering me cigarettes. He says they can really help to take the edge off things. Can't I have just one, once in a while?

Answer: Your friend may be trying to help, but you need to find a healthier way to deal with stress.

Just the way you phrased your question shows how a habit can begin, moving from "just one" to "once in a while." From there, it moves on to "one a day" and up to "a pack a day" and even more.

DID YOU KNOW?

Percentage of Adult Smokers by State, 2006

State	Adult Smokers	State	Adult Smokers
Alabama	23.3%	Montana	19.0%
Alaska	24.2%	Nebraska	18.6%
Arizona	18.1%	Nevada	22.2%
Arkansas	23.7%	New Hampshire	18.7%
California	14.9%	New Jersey	18.1%
Colorado	17.9%	New Mexico	20.2%
Connecticut	17.0%	New York	18.3%
Delaware	21.7%	North Carolina	22.1%
D.C.	17.9%	North Dakota	19.6%
Florida	21.0%	Ohio	22.5%
Georgia	20.0%	Oklahoma	25.1%
Hawaii	17.5%	Oregon	18.5%
Idaho	16.8%	Pennsylvania	21.5%
Illinois	20.5%	Rhode Island	19.3%
Indiana	24.1%	South Carolina	22.3%
Iowa	21.5%	South Dakota	20.4%
Kansas	20.0%	Tennessee	22.6%
Kentucky	28.6%	Texas	18.1%
Louisiana	23.4%	Utah	9.8%
Maine	20.9%	Vermont	18.0%
Maryland	17.8%	Virginia	19.3%
Massachusetts	17.8%	Washington	17.1%
Michigan	22.4%	West Virginia	25.7%
Minnesota	18.3%	Wisconsin	20.8%
Mississippi	25.1%	Wyoming	21.6%
Missouri	23.3%		

The percentage of people who smoke varies by state. Utah has the lowest percentage of smokers, at 9.8 percent. Kentucky has the highest percentage of smokers, at 28.6 percent. States that produce tobacco products have a higher percentage of residents that smoke.

Source: Centers for Disease Control, 2006

DIFFERENCES IN SMOKING BY AGE

Most smokers—19.6 million—are between 25 and 44 years old. This high rate is due in part to a rise in teen smoking back in the 1990s. The smallest adult number—3.0 million—is smokers over age 65. A grim reason for that last statistic might be that many smokers have died before that age. For the youngest adult category, ages 18–24, the Lung Association finds 6.8 million smokers. Below that age, the **Centers for Disease Control and Prevention** (CDC) estimates that there are an additional three million smokers in the 12–17 age range. For antismoking activists, these last two groups are critical. Of all smokers, over 90 percent began before the age of 21.

INTO THE FUTURE

Tobacco's voyage around the world started more than 500 years ago and continues today. Instead of spreading haphazardly with wandering people, however, the product's growth is controlled by giant corporations driven by market forces.

Health concerns, regulations, and antismoking activism and education have reduced smoking in the United States and developed countries in northern and western Europe. In response, tobacco companies are finding new markets, new profits, and millions of new smokers among the nations of eastern Europe and worldwide among developing countries.

See also: Government and Tobacco; Smoking and Society; Tobacco Worldwide

FURTHER READING

Gately, Iain. *Tobacco.* New York: Grove Press, 2002.
Goel, Rajeev K., and Michael A. Nelson. *Global Efforts to Combat Smoking.* Burlington, Vt.: Ashgate, 2008.

■ SMOKELESS TOBACCO

See: Tobacco Products

■ SOCIAL SMOKING

See: Peer Pressure and Smoking; Smoking and Society

■ SPORTS AND SMOKING

From the early days of cigarette production, tobacco companies liked to portray their products as good, healthy fun. What better way than to connect cigarettes with athletes?

Tobacco companies made this connection early by creating the first baseball cards. Pictures of players were printed on the cardboard sheets that stiffened cigarette packs. A 1909 set featured Pittsburgh Pirates star Honus Wagner, a nonsmoker who objected to having his picture used to advertise cigarettes, especially since the cards were collected by children. He demanded that his card be destroyed, ironically creating one of the great collector's items of all time. In 2000, a surviving Honus Wagner card sold for more than a million dollars.

Until the 1960s, tobacco companies often featured sports stars in their advertisements. Even today, cigarette ads in magazines often show smokers playing Frisbee, softball, or football.

TEENS SPEAK

I Was a Secondhand Sports Smoker

Dan is 20 years old, a junior in college. He started smoking when he was 15.

"My older brother was a real racing fan. He loved to go to the speedway, and he was always coming back with stuff. Baseball caps, jackets, they all had the logo for a brand of cigarettes. Sometimes he even came home with packs of cigarettes—freebies. They'd hand them out as samples.

"I was a big kid—played a little football. The hats and jackets fit me. One day, I tried my brother's cigarettes on for size too. He and my folks were pretty mad, but I didn't think it was such a big deal. Hey, if all those famous racers were involved, smoking couldn't be all that bad.

These days, almost any sport moves are too fast for me to play. I just can't catch my breath. About the best I can do is a nice, slow game of softball.

"When it comes to sports, I guess I'm a spectator. Of course, that makes it easier to light up during a game. But now that I'm driving over to the speedway, I notice they're not giving cigarettes away anymore."

WHERE DOES THE MEDIA STAND?

Both the print and broadcast media are money-making businesses. Cigarette advertisements featuring sports stars brought profits to newspapers, magazines, radio and television stations and, of course, tobacco companies. Unless pressured by public opinion or legal action, media companies have generally shown themselves unwilling to forgo a lucrative source of advertising money.

Continuing criticism over the use of prominent sports figures to sell cigarettes resulted in a 1963 agreement by tobacco companies to discontinue promotion by sports stars. In 1971, Congress banned TV ads for cigarettes. Cigarette manufacturers quickly found a new way to get their brand names on television. They sponsored sporting events. The Marlboro name quickly became attached to auto racing, as did Winston and Skoal, a smokeless tobacco. Virginia Slims sponsored tennis tournaments.

Researchers from the Boston University School of Public Health studied the events sponsored by tobacco corporations between 1995 and 1999. In that five-year span, the companies attached their names not only to a variety of sporting events but also to musical and cultural performances and social causes. Motor racing received the highest promotional expenditure, with more than $208 million going to various organizations and events. Besides racing and tennis, major tobacco sponsorships involved rodeo, golf, and pool playing. One company donated $3 million to help complete the construction of a university football stadium.

Some tobacco companies came up with clever marketing connections for sports. For example, Philip Morris used billboard space inside sports arenas to ensure that the company's Marlboro ads were placed wherever TV game coverage was likely to focus. Marlboro billboards appeared behind the goal posts in football stadiums and over the team entrances to the field. The TV networks caught these silent ads in their cameras. It took government action—a suit by the U.S. Justice Department in 1995—to end the practice.

Fact Or Fiction?

I see some people are making a big deal out of sports stars using smokeless tobacco. Don't these guys have a right to a private life?

The Facts: Being in the public eye means losing much of one's privacy. Like it or not, sports figures are role models. They are cheered by countless young fans who will even pay for the opportunity of getting an autograph. These young people practice throwing a pass or swinging a bat like their hero. They also try out their hero's habits.

When baseball players began using smokeless tobacco in televised games, the youth rate didn't double, triple, or even quadruple. According to a report by the Centers for Disease Control and Prevention, the rate shot up to eight times the original number of users in 10 years. That is a serious demonstration, both of the reach of the media and the strength of hero worship.

WHERE DOES NASCAR STAND?

The sport of stock car racing began in the hills of North Carolina—tobacco country. Early support for the National Association for Stock Car Auto Racing (NASCAR) came from tobacco companies. R.J. Reynolds (RJR) was among the first to associate one of its brand names, Winston, with NASCAR racing.

Beginning in 1971, the company sponsored NASCAR short-track racing events as well as the high-prestige Winston Cup racing series. These races got considerable television coverage, putting the Winston name in millions of homes. Philip Morris supported a racing team whose cars were plastered with Marlboro logos. The Skoal Bandit became another rolling advertisement, this time for smokeless tobacco.

Although NASCAR took some criticism, the arrangement continued. RJR and the racing association signed a series of five-year contracts. RJR was spending $60 million a year to promote the sport, recruit sponsors for race teams, and improve racing tracks. Tobacco money turned NASCAR into the nation's number one spectator sport. In return, those spectators were invited to sample Winstons or trade in their current brand for four packs of Winstons.

The first major problem came in 1999, after the Master Settlement Agreement (MSA), an out-of-court settlement that ended a lawsuit between the tobacco companies and state governments. Although the main thrust of the case was repayment for state health-care costs associated with tobacco-related diseases, the agreement also included new restrictions on tobacco advertising and promotion, especially involving young people. The MSA prohibited cigarette companies from sponsoring sporting events with competitors under the age of 18. Some of the NASCAR short-track races allowed drivers as young as 16.

Although NASCAR racing drew the second largest audience in televised sports, NASCAR officials now found themselves limited in promotion. Winston was not allowed to use its affiliation with the races in radio or TV ads. Officials wanted racing to enter the mainstream. As early as 1998, RJR invited NASCAR to consider alternatives. In 2003, the racing association reached an agreement with Nextel, a giant wireless telephone company. If you look on the NASCAR web site, you'll find logos for three racing series, sponsored by Nextel, Busch beer, and Craftsman tools.

Q & A

Question: I'd never smoke—I play sports, and smoking ruins your wind. But some guys say smokeless tobacco actually helps your game. Is that true?

Answer: Some athletes think that smokeless tobacco gives them extra energy, but what they're feeling is the product's powerful nicotine rush. A 1995 study of Major League baseball players published in the *Journal of the American Dental Association* found that a player's performance—batting, fielding, or pitching—was not affected by smokeless tobacco.

In a 1998 study published in *Medicine & Science in Sports & Exercise,* researchers tested reaction time and strength of two groups of college athletes. One group used smokeless tobacco. The other used no tobacco products at all. The results showed that smokeless tobacco use had no effect on reaction time. However, the product may have reduced the strength of the athletes who used it.

You'll play better—and stay healthier—if you keep away from all forms of tobacco.

WHERE DOES BASEBALL STAND?

Baseball was invented in the mid-1800s, a time when most American tobacco users chewed rather than smoked. When the National League was organized in 1876, cigarettes were still rolled by hand. Even when the American League came along in 1901, cigarettes were just beginning to become popular.

Many early ball players came from southern or rural states where chewing tobacco was popular. Also, having a "chaw" in one's mouth was useful. Chewing tobacco kept the mouth moist while playing on hot, open fields under the summer sun. Spit was also useful in keeping the players' leather gloves pliable. Some players found chewing tobacco to be a useful tool in the days of the spitball, a pitch that was banned from baseball in 1920. By the 1930s and 1940s, however, most players smoked cigarettes.

As the dangers of smoking became news in the 1970s, some ball players switched to what they believed was a safer form of tobacco. Players first went to chewing tobacco, then started dipping snuff, holding a pinch of powdered tobacco between the lip and the gums. Chewing tobacco and snuff companies began marketing their products as "smokeless tobacco." Part of their promotional efforts, as noted in a 1992 article in the *Journal of Public Health,* involved sending free samples to major league, minor league, and even college baseball teams.

By the 1980s, smokeless tobacco (or spit tobacco, as it's called by antismoking activists) was widespread in the major leagues. Players used spit tobacco on televised games, giving free air time to a product that was banned from advertising on TV. Analysis of Game Four of the 1986 World Series showed that players spent 23 minutes using spit tobacco—essentially a free advertisement for the product in the middle of one of the nation's most popular sporting events. By contrast, during the same game in 2002, players spent only five minutes using smokeless tobacco on camera.

On the whole, promotion of smokeless tobacco was very successful. According to a 1993 report by the Centers for Disease Control and Prevention between 1972 and 1991 consumption of smokeless tobacco products tripled in the United States. In that same period, eight times as many 17- to 19-year-olds started the habit. Young people still make up an important segment of spit tobacco sales.

Former players who recognized the dangers of smokeless tobacco formed NSTEP, the National Spit Tobacco Education Program, in 1994. Among these players was Bob Tuttle, a former star for the Minnesota Twins, who underwent disfiguring cancer surgery because of his spit tobacco habit. Joe Garagiola, a former player and sportscaster, lost a tobacco-chewing friend to cancer. Garagiola took the lead in sounding the alarm about the dangers of smokeless tobacco. "You lose one

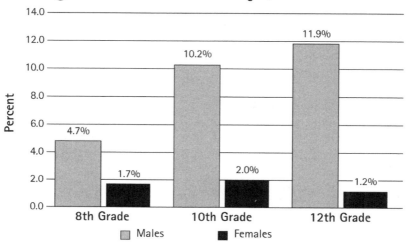

DID YOU KNOW?

Percentage of 8th, 10th, and 12th Graders Who Reported Using Smokeless Tobacco During the Previous 30 Days, 2007

As the chart shows, male adolescents are more likely than females to use smokeless tobacco. The 2007 estimates are approximately half of the peak levels of smokeless tobacco use found during the mid 1990s. However, the percentage of 8th, 10th, and 12th graders using smokeless tobacco has been relatively stable since 2002.

Source: National Institutes on Drug Abuse, "The Monitoring the Future: Overview of Key Findings," 2007.

piece of your face at a time until you are dead," Garagiola warned today's players.

NSTEP sponsors a yearly mouth examination of minor league players by dentists. In 2001, of the 2,000 players examined, 300 had sores in their mouths from smokeless tobacco use, and in 21 cases, those sores were cancerous or precancerous.

Major League Baseball, the players' union, and the team trainers' organization support NSTEP's goals. When the organization started working with Major League Baseball in 1998, 38.5 percent of major leaguers admitted using smokeless tobacco. By 2002, that number had dropped to 30.5 percent.

Although some teams ban players in uniform from carrying snuff or chewing tobacco, they can't stop players from using the product on the field without negotiating the issue with the players' union. Spit tobacco is banned from the minor leagues, though many minor league players admit to using smokeless products. In 1994, the National Collegiate Athletic Association (NCAA), the major organization for college sports, banned all tobacco products. However, a 2001 NCAA survey found 41 percent of college baseball players and 28.9 percent of football players still using smokeless tobacco.

A STRONG SELLING TEAM

Sports and sports figures have long been a part of selling and promoting tobacco products. For years, sports stars endorsed cigarettes and chewing tobacco, even though they may later have suffered as a result of using the products. Joe DiMaggio and Babe Ruth were famous players who appeared in tobacco ads. Both died from tobacco-related illnesses. DiMaggio, a smoker, died of lung cancer. Ruth, who smoked and also chewed tobacco from the age of seven, died of throat cancer.

Sponsorship of sporting events became a successful tactic for tobacco promotion, especially after the 1971 ban on television advertising for cigarettes. In recent years, however, some sports groups have reconsidered their connections to tobacco. NASCAR racing officials finally cut a long-standing relationship with Winston cigarettes, and Major League Baseball has begun efforts to ban tobacco products. However, many individual athletes have not ended—or been able to end—their tobacco habits.

See also: Advertising and Smoking; Media and Smoking, The; Tobacco Products

FURTHER READING
Gately, Iain. *Tobacco*. New York: Grove Press, 2002.
Haugen, David M. *How Does Advertising Impact Teen Behavior?* Farmington Hills, Mich.: Greenhaven Press, 2008.
Penncock, Angela E. *Advertising Sin and Sickness: The Politics of Alcohol and Tobacco Marketing, 1950–1990.* Dekalb: Northern Illinois Press, 2007.

■ TOBACCO AS A GATEWAY PRODUCT

"Monitoring the Future," sponsored by the National Institute on Drug Abuse (NIDA), is an annual survey of more than 40,000 students. The survey collects information on student drug use and attitudes. The 2007 survey showed that 18.8 percent of 12th graders used marijuana in the last 30 days, 3.7 percent used amphetamines, and 1.3 percent used Ecstasy. More than 44 percent had used alcohol in the last 30 days, and 12.3 percent smoked on a daily basis.

The inclusion of tobacco and alcohol among the substances used to introduce people to illegal drugs explains the term *gateway product*. Tobacco and alcohol are legal—at least for adults. However, given their addictive and damaging properties, if either had been recently discovered, the Food and Drug Administration (FDA) would undoubtedly ban them as dangerous.

Tobacco and alcohol are also the most easily obtained addictive and brain-altering substances for most teenagers. They are easily available at supermarkets, convenience stores, or gas stations. All that teens need is money and a fake ID or a negligent or accommodating store clerk. What an underage person learns while trying to buy a six-pack or a carton of cigarettes is essentially how to buy illegal drugs.

TEENS SPEAK

What Drugs?

Celia is a petite, 17-year-old junior in high school. She's been smoking for two years.

"We were asked to fill out a questionnaire not too long ago. It was anonymous, so everybody could give honest answers. At least I thought we were giving honest answers.

"One of the questions was about whether I'd used any gateway drugs. I thought they were talking about marijuana, so I said 'no.'"

She rolls her eyes and giggles. "Then they gave us the follow-up class session, and a whole bunch of us got a shock. Guess what? Gateway drugs included cigarettes and alcohol. I've done both, and I know a lot of my friends have too.

"My dad smokes, and he always keeps a carton of cigarettes on his dresser. Sometimes he has business in the next state where cigarette prices are lower. Then he'll come back with a couple of cartons and stash the extra one in the cellar. We've got a bunch of shelves down there with extra food supplies. When I was a kid, we'd play store down there.

She rolls her eyes again. "That's where I had my first taste of beer—warm beer, from off the shelves. It was pretty disgusting. We used to smoke some of dad's extra cigarettes down there, till the smell gave us away. Busted," she laughs, then grows more serious. "Busted for drugs."

DISTURBING NUMBERS

It seems reasonable to assume that trying one illicit product might lead to similar experimentation with stronger substances. After all, a person can't even smoke marijuana until he or she has mastered the mechanics of the cigarette—inhaling smoke and keeping it in the lungs. Are there any facts to back up such assumptions? Statistics on the connection between gateway substances and illegal drugs are numerous and daunting.

In 1986, NIDA released the results of a 10–year study of student attitudes about alcohol and tobacco. According to that research, 18.4 percent of high school seniors who smoked also drank daily, compared to a drinking rate of 1.7 percent among nonsmoking seniors. Nearly 68 percent of the seniors who smoked drank heavily, while only 17.2 percent of nonsmoking seniors engaged in heavy drinking.

The December 1990 issue of the *American Health Journal*, confirmed those findings with the results of another NIDA study. This survey found that 12- to 17-year-olds who smoked cigarettes were 14 times more likely to abuse alcohol, 100 times more likely to smoke marijuana, and 32 times more likely to use cocaine than their nonsmoking peers.

A 1994 study by Columbia University's Center on Addiction and Substance Abuse (CASA) also commented on gateway drugs. Based on a survey of 30,000 American households, the researchers found that nearly 90 percent of cocaine users either smoked tobacco, drank alcoholic beverages, or used marijuana first. Young smokers were found to be 19 times more likely to use cocaine than nonsmokers. They were also found to be 13 times more likely to use heroin than young people who did not smoke.

The Centers for Disease Control and Prevention (CDC) reported in 1995 that teenagers who smoked were three times more likely than nonsmokers to use alcohol, eight times more likely to use marijuana, and 22 times more likely to use cocaine.

In a 2007 report by CASA, researchers found that teenagers between the ages of 12 and 17 who currently smoke are five times more likely to drink than nonsmoking teens. The researchers also found that teenagers who currently smoke are 8.5 times more likely than nonsmoking teens to use illicit drugs. Teens who smoke are 13.4 times more likely than nonsmoking teens to use marijuana.

A report by Columbia University's Center on Addiction and Substance Abuse found that in 2007, smokers 12- to 17-year-old are more than 8.5 times as likely to use illicit drugs.

A 1996 study detailed in the *Journal of Addictive Diseases* showed that 90 percent of alcoholics were also smokers. The habit is three times more widespread among alcoholics than among the general population. Similar research done by NIDA in 2000 showed that 66 percent of drug users also smoked. In this case, the smoking rate was more than twice that of the general population.

The web of dependencies is complicated and not easy to follow. However, the connections are strong and can easily be found.

Fact Or Fiction?

This "gateway drug" stuff is blown way out of proportion. It's just kids acting up.

The Facts: A number of knowledgeable people in the health field take tobacco smoking much more seriously than mere "acting up." In 1988, the surgeon general, the government's most senior public health official, issued a report entitled "The Health Consequences of Smoking: Nicotine Addiction." This report found that the nicotine in tobacco is a psychoactive drug, a substance that affects the brain and the mind, altering the user's mood. Nicotine's physical and psychological effects are compared with cocaine, heroin, and also alcohol. Young people who experiment with cigarettes are flirting with addiction and opening the door to other addictive experiences.

TRYING ON TROUBLE

The mountain of statistics on the progression from gateway substances to harder drugs does not mean that everyone who takes a puff on a cigarette—or a sip from a beer can—will end up a helpless cocaine addict. However, a troubling percentage of young people who experiment with alcohol and tobacco do graduate to more potent and dangerous substances.

Consuming alcohol and tobacco can have serious consequences, both in the long term and the short term. Tobacco can lead to cancer, respiratory ailments, and cardiovascular disease. Drinking has its own set of unhealthful and dangerous results.

Several government agencies are attempting to keep statistics on young people and the dangerous or unhealthy things they do. The CDC runs the Youth Risk Behavior Surveillance System, asking seventh- through 12th-graders questions about everything from drinking to suicide. The National Institute of Child Health and Human Development (NICHD) commissioned the 1995 National Survey of Adolescent Males, a long-term study following young men from their teen years into adulthood. The NICHD and 17 other federal agencies funded the National Longitudinal Study of Adolescent Health in 1994.

To gain an overall picture of the ways young people endanger themselves, the Department of Health and Human Services commissioned an analysis of the results from all three of surveys in 2000. "Teen Risk-Taking: A Statistical Portrait" examined 10 major forms of risky behavior found in all the government surveys, with an emphasis on multiple risk taking.

The study found that, in general, 54 percent of the respondents engaged in some form of risky behavior. As the grade levels went higher, so did the percentage of risk-taking teens. Only 19 percent of seventh- and eighth-graders engaged in multiple risks. That percentage grew to 36 percent of high school juniors and seniors. A small percentage—4 percent—engaged in five or more risky activities.

Only 11 percent of the respondents were smokers. Out of that group, however, 85 percent took other risks: regular alcohol use, 35 percent; regular binge drinking, 40 percent; marijuana smoking, 35 percent; use of other drugs, 41 percent; fighting, 17 percent; carrying weapons, 21 percent; suicidal thoughts, 19 percent; suicide attempts, 24 percent; engaging in unprotected sexual intercourse, 25 percent.

Many young people start smoking to look "experienced." As this study shows, they may discover that they've opened the door to more experiences than they really want.

Q & A

Question: Louie was my best friend growing up, but now he's hanging with a bunch of guys who smoke. How can I stay friendly with him when he wants to get me in with his new crew?

Answer: You do not have to drop a friend because he starts smoking. Just make sure his new friends don't insist that you have to smoke to hang out together.

If everybody is expected to smoke, be aware that this is a big decision. Don't make it lightly. And let your friend know that he'll also have to make an important choice, between his smoking buddies and his best friend.

See also: Alcohol and Tobacco Use; Drugs and Tobacco Abuse

FURTHER READING

Abrams, David B., Raymond Niaura, Richard A. Brown, Karen M. Emmons, Michael G. Goldstein, Peter M. Monti, and Laura A. Linnan. *The Tobacco Dependence Treatment Handbook: A Guide to Best Practices.* New York: Guilford Press, 2003.

Alters, Sandra M. *Alcohol, Tobacco, and Illicit Drugs.* Farmington, Mich.: Information Plus Reference Series, 2007.

Bellenir, Karen, ed. *Substance Abuse Sourcebook.* Detroit: Omnigraphics, 1996.

■ TOBACCO PRODUCTS

The main tobacco products are pipe tobacco, snuff, chewing tobacco, cigars, and cigarettes. Today, with pipe smokers making up only a small percentage of tobacco users, the other forms of tobacco dominate the market.

SNUFF

Snuff is powdered tobacco that is either snorted up into the nose or "dipped," held in a wad between the lower lip and the gums. Snuff has been around for hundreds of years. In the days before machine manufacturing, snuff was very expensive to produce. In the 1600s and 1700s, it was used mainly by the wealthy.

Inhaled snuff delivers **nicotine**, the addictive ingredient of tobacco, to the body through the nasal membranes, the damp skin within the nose. Taking snuff by mouth allows nicotine to pass through the moist skin of the inner lips and gums. Although many users believe "smokeless" tobacco is safer than smoking, they're wrong. Researchers have found 28 cancer-causing chemicals in dip tobacco.

In addition, one can of snuff has as much nicotine as 60 cigarettes. Blood tests of those who use smokeless tobacco revealed twice as much nicotine in their blood compared to cigarette smokers. The nicotine dose is so high that smokeless tobacco companies offer "junior brands" for those starting the habit. The amount of nicotine in the regular brands would make new users sick. The high nicotine doses also cause difficulty for smokeless tobacco users who attempt to quit.

CHEW

In 1900, chewing tobacco was the most popular tobacco product in the United States. Made of shredded tobacco, it is sold in moist cakes, plugs, or in twists. When held between the gums and the cheek, chewing tobacco delivers nicotine through the skin inside the mouth.

While chewing tobacco is much less common than it was a century ago, the product has been making a comeback. Along with dip, it's often used by baseball players to keep the mouth moist on hot, dry ball fields. This much-publicized use of the product, plus heightened advertising, has convinced some young people that smokeless tobacco is a safe alternative to smoking. One study found that while 77 percent of students consider smoking dangerous, only 40 percent worried about smokeless tobacco.

Unfortunately, chewing tobacco has the same cancer-causing chemicals as snuff. Other unhealthy ingredients include formaldehyde, a poisonous chemical used to preserve dead flesh, and poisonous metals like cadmium and lead.

One of the less attractive behaviors connected with chewing tobacco is the continual need to spit out the brownish saliva that accumulates in the mouth. Swallowing can make users sick. When the chewing habit was popular a hundred years ago, public places had spittoons—spit buckets—for collecting this tobacco byproduct.

CIGARS

Cigars—chopped tobacco wrapped in tobacco leaves—were popular in the 1800s. In the 1990s, they made a comeback, with many celebrities taking up the habit. As a film star, Arnold Schwarzenegger made large, expensive cigars part of his public image, smoking them on interview shows while promoting his movies. The better brands of cigars can be very expensive, so they have the reputation of being a status smoke. An upscale magazine, *Cigar Aficionado*, discusses costly brands that cost $10 each.

Less expensive cigars are also smoked in the United States. The CDC for 2005 found that 14 percent of American high school students tried cigars in the month before the survey. The figures came to 19.2 percent for boys and 18.7 percent for girls.

Besides their celebrity boost, cigars have generally not received as much adverse publicity as cigarettes. Many people believe cigars are less dangerous because the smoke is not inhaled into the lungs.

Unfortunately, cigar smoking still poses serious health risks. Statistically, male cigar smokers are about 33 percent more likely to develop cancer than nonsmokers. According to the American Cancer Society, cigar smokers have a particular risk of cancer to the mouth, esophagus (throat), and larynx (voicebox). Their chances of developing these diseases are four to 10 times greater than nonsmokers.

CIGARETTES

Cigarettes—chopped tobacco rolled in paper—are the major tobacco product in the United States. In 2006, 371 billion cigarettes were smoked in the United State.

Because of the large numbers (and the large amounts of money) involved, the battle over cigarette smoking remains the focus of efforts to control the use of tobacco.

Throughout the 1990s, secret documents from tobacco companies became public through leaks or as a result of legal action. Among these is a memo from Brown & Williamson, one of the large cigarette makers. While the paper discusses the company's five-year operating cycle through 1998, it mentions that the cost of producing a pack of cigarettes was 19 cents—less than a penny per cigarette. Tobacco giant R.J. Reynolds reports that it costs $1.38 to produce a pack of cigarettes, while New York State's Quitline argues it only costs five cents to produce each pack. R.J. Reynolds also states that the company makes a $.24 profit for each pack of cigarettes they sell.

As long as tobacco companies can pass along this amount—which is small, compared to most retail cigarette prices—cigarettes will remain a profitable business.

Q & A

Question: The tobacco companies call it "smokeless tobacco." Why do the antitobacco people call it "spit tobacco?"

Answer: Calling the product "smokeless tobacco" is a marketing ploy. It makes this tobacco sound safer and cleaner. Calling it "spit tobacco" points out what happens in a dipper's mouth. The tobacco mixes with saliva. This mixture can stain clothes, damage teeth and gums, cause cancer, and still needs to be spit out, as viewers have seen baseball players do on the field for years.

TRENDS: THE RISE OF SMOKELESS TOBACCO

The official internet site for the U.S. Smokeless Tobacco Company, maker of such brands as Skoal and Copenhagan snuff, describes the company as "the leading producer and marketer of the only growing segment of the U.S. tobacco industry." Where other tobacco products face declining sales, smokeless tobacco continues to expand.

In the 1970s, snuff and chewing tobacco were used mainly by older men, 65 years of age and up. The decade of the 1970s was also a time of heightened concern about the dangers of cigarette smoke. Some smokers began using chewing tobacco as a way to get their nicotine without inhaling. Always quick to take advantage of a trend, the snuff and chew manufacturers renamed their products "smokeless tobacco" and began promoting them heavily.

The continuing tradition of oral tobacco in baseball offered the industry high-profile users. Throughout the 1980s, use of the products soared. Between 1972 and 1991, consumption of smokeless tobacco products tripled in the United States. By 1991, eight times as many 17- to 19-year-olds used smokeless tobacco compared to users of the same age in 1972. According to the 2006 National Survey on Drug Use and

Health, an estimated 8.2 million Americans used smokeless tobacco. "Monitoring the Future," an annual health survey of young people, found in 2007 that 6.6 percent of high school seniors used smokeless tobacco in the last 30 days.

Is it better for you?

Smokeless tobacco manufacturers claim that use of their product is safer than smoking. Users don't draw poisonous smoke into their lungs, so there is no threat of lung cancer. This suggestion seemed to have a deep impression on teens. In a 2007 study in *Nicotine and Tobacco Research*, investigators found that 89.3 percent of college freshmen believed smokeless tobacco was just as, or more, harmful than cigarettes. This means that 10.7 percent thought smokeless tobacco was less harmful than cigarettes. Obviously the overwhelming majority of college freshmen disagree with the tobacco industry's claim that smokeless tobacco is less harmful than smoking.

"Safer" does not necessarily mean "safe," as even proponents of smokeless tobacco admit. There are still serious problems with smokeless tobacco, including the risk of cancer.

Health consequences

Doctors diagnose oral cancer in approximately 34,000 Americans each year. About 75 percent of those cases can be traced to tobacco, either smoked or smokeless. According to the American Cancer Society, almost one-half of the people diagnosed (46 percent) will be dead within five years. In nearly 70 percent of cases, the cancer has spread to lymph nodes—and possibly farther through the body—by the time a diagnosis is made.

In comparison, approximately 213,380 new cases of lung cancer are expected in 2007. Although there is less risk of cancer, smokeless tobacco users are still endangering their health. While more Americans end up with lung cancer than oral cancer, death rates for oral cancer haven't really improved in 30 years, and oral cancers often metastasize before they're discovered.

Smokeless tobacco users should be aware of the warning signs of oral cancer. Sores are a common problem for smokeless tobacco users. However, a sore that bleeds easily and doesn't heal—or a red or white patch in the mouth that doesn't go away—is a cause for concern. The white sores are called leukoplakia, and they're a precancerous condition. Other signs to be aware of include a lump or thickening anywhere in the mouth, soreness or swelling that doesn't go away, or trouble chewing, swallowing, or moving the tongue or jaw.

While good health calls for most people to visit the dentist twice a year, smokeless tobacco users are urged to go every three months for safety's sake. Early detection of oral cancer boosts chances of surviving.

Dealing with oral cancer means surgery, which can be disfiguring. Unless the cancer is caught early, surgeons have to take out large sections of the mouth, tongue, or jaw.

Although Congress acted in 1967 to place warnings on packs of cigarettes, it was not until 1986 that President Ronald Reagan signed into law a bill requiring a similar warning label on smokeless tobacco packages. Actually, buyers may find one of three possible labels. One warns of oral cancer, another of gum disease and tooth loss, while the third tells users that the product is not a safe alternative to cigarettes.

Lower on the danger scale but still of concern are the effects of smokeless tobacco on the teeth and gums. Nicotine and other chemicals in smokeless tobacco irritate the tissues in the mouth, resulting in bleeding gums and sores, receding gums, gum disease, and lost teeth. Also, users of smokeless tobacco soak their teeth in spit laced with sugar used to flavor the tobacco, leading to tooth decay.

A hidden addiction?

Medical tests have shown that smokeless tobacco users carry a much higher dose of nicotine in their blood, even compared to cigarette smoker's. Living with a higher dose of any drug means the user's addiction is stronger. Ironically, boosters of smokeless tobacco like to compare it to nicotine replacement gums—users can enjoy it in places where they are not permitted to smoke. The gum, however, is supposed to get smokers *out* of the nicotine habit, not push them deeper into it.

Reports about office use of smokeless tobacco have not just reached the ears of cancer researchers. A March 22, 2004, issue of the *Charlotte Observer* carried a story about smokeless tobacco product, the first that does not require the user to spit. It consists of powdered tobacco inside a tiny paper package. The article reports that although many disliked the new product, one user described it enthusiastically as "just the thing for a nicotine fit in a nonsmoking environment!"

TRENDS AND FUTURE PRODUCTS

Tobacco companies are test-marketing and even introducing a range of new products. R.J. Reynolds's Eclipse cigarette has a carbon rod inside the cigarette that heats rather than burns the tobacco. The smoke contains fewer chemicals created by combustion and is supposed to be less harmful.

Are they safer?

Each of the companies making claims that its products are safe provides the results of tests. Some were conducted in-house and others by independent laboratories.

Antismoking proponents, however, remember the 1950s, a time when cigarette manufacturers made extravagant claims about the health benefits of filtered cigarettes.

They also remember the last wave of tobacco innovation—the low-tar, low-nicotine brands introduced in the 1970s. The government tested these "light" cigarettes on special smoking machines. When the machines registered lower levels of dangerous materials, millions of consumers switched to these new, supposedly healthier cigarettes. Unfortunately, humans don't smoke the way machines do. Since they weren't getting the amount of nicotine they were used to from the new cigarettes, smokers puffed much harder on them, defeating the purpose of the filters. In fact, smokers actually inhaled more smoke—and tar—much deeper into their lungs.

It took years for the bad effects to become obvious. The episode shows that even when the government tries to come up with an objective test for cigarettes, it does not always succeed.

New nicotine products

In recent years, many smokers have successfully quit the habit with the help of nicotine replacement therapy, receiving doses of nicotine through patches, gum, nasal sprays, and lozenges. Several companies have tried to cash in on this success by marketing new nicotine products; these items have not been tested as drugs to help people stop smoking.

In 2002, the Food and Drug Administration banned the sale of nicotine lip salve and nicotine lollipops. These nicotine-replacement products contained chemicals that had not been tested for safety.

THE OLD AND THE NEW

Some tobacco products have existed in recognizable form for hundreds of years, perhaps for thousands. In all that time, people have shown considerable ingenuity in coming up with new varieties of tobacco that offer improved taste or a stronger effect. Driven by the profit motive, large corporations have accelerated the effort, inventing some tobacco products that seem completely novel. However, the one characteristic that links all of these products is that they present in one degree or another a health risk for users. Only time will tell if there are any dangers in the new products entering the market.

See also: Sports and Smoking

FURTHER READING

Alters, Sandra M. *Alcohol, Tobacco, and Illicit Drugs.* Farmington, Mich.: Information Plus Reference Series, 2007.
Gately, Iain. *Tobacco.* New York: Grove Press, 2002.
Whetherall, Charles. *Quit: Read This Book and Stop Smoking.* Philadelphia: Running Press Miniature Editions, 2007.

■ TOBACCO USE AND SOCIOECONOMIC GROUPS

Class differences in smoking habits. Society is made up of different socioeconomic groups, usually referred to as social classes. Broadly speaking, there are the upper classes, middle classes, and lower classes. The difference between classes is based traditionally on level of education, income, and job prestige. In general, these factors make up a person's socioeconomic status.

Studies show that tobacco use differs by socioeconomic status. Members of a lower socioeconomic status are more likely to start and continue smoking. They are also less likely to try smoking-cessation programs. Tobacco companies understand this and actively market to the lower classes, which they refer to as the downscale market.

SOCIOECONOMIC STATUS
AND SMOKING BEHAVIORS

Socioeconomic status generally refers to a person's position in society. People with high incomes and/or advanced educational degrees are viewed as more successful than others. Often people think about socioeconomic status in terms of the "haves" and the "have-nots." The assumption is that "the haves" possess the skills or opportunities necessary to succeed in life. From a social and economic standpoint, they are viewed as "better-off" than members of lower socioeconomic groups.

The Centers for Disease Control and Prevention (CDC) estimate that 20.8 percent of U.S. adults actively smoked in 2006. The prevalence of smoking varied by both education and income. Smoking was most prevalent among people who earned a GED (46 percent), a high school diploma (24 percent), or never graduated from high school (27 percent). These figures are significantly higher when compared to the number of college graduates who smoke. The CDC found that only 9.6 percent of college graduates actively smoked. College graduates were between 2.5 and five times *less* likely to smoke than those with lower levels of education.

In a 2003 study in the *Journal of Epidemiology and Community Health*, authors found that people with lower socioeconomic status were more likely to start smoking and become regular smokers. More than 90 percent of people with less than a high school diploma admitted to smoking at some point in their lives. Almost 95 percent of this group became active smokers. Only 82 percent of people with a high school diploma ever tried smoking, with almost 85 percent of them becoming active smokers. The numbers drop significantly for college-educated people, with 66 percent of them ever smoking. Only 49 percent of this group became active smokers.

Q & A

Question: Does a parent's socioeconomic status influence an adolescent's likelihood of smoking?

Answer: In a 2003 study in the *Journal of Epidemiology and Community Health,* researchers looked at parents' socioeconomic status to see if it influenced their children's likelihood of smoking. They found that parental socioeconomic status did influence the likelihood of children smoking. Children who lived in poverty between birth and seven years of age were more likely to smoke as adults than children who did not live in poverty early in their lives. In particular, a mother's level of education influenced the likelihood of a child's becoming a regular smoker. The lower a mother's education, the greater the odds of her children becoming smokers.

In a 2003 study in the *American Journal of Public Health,* authors also found that adolescent smoking was influenced by their parents' socioeconomic status. For example, when parents did not complete high school, adolescents were 28 percent more likely to smoke than those whose parents graduated high school (but did not go on to college). Adolescents were 30 percent more likely to smoke when their parents earned less than $20,000 per year when compared to those whose presents earned between $20,000 and $30,000.

In a 2007 study in the *American Journal of Public Health*, researchers found that young adults (ages 18–24) without a college education smoked at more than twice the rate of young adults with a college education. Approximately 33 percent of young adults smoke if they do not have a college education. This compares to only 14 percent of young adults who smoke and have a college education.

In a 2004 study in the *American Journal of Public Health*, authors found that current smoking behavior was highest among those with less education, less income, and those who worked in service or blue collar jobs. In particular, the odds of being a current smoker was highest for people whose income was less than 200 percent of the poverty line. The odds of current smoking were also highest for people who, at most, had a GED or high school diploma.

SOCIOECONOMIC STATUS AND SMOKING CESSATION

Socioeconomic status also influences the ability to quit smoking. In a 2003 study in the *Journal of Epidemiology and Community Health,* researchers discovered that socioeconomic status influenced smoking cessation. Only 8.3 percent of regular smokers with less than a high school diploma stopped smoking. This compares to 54.6 percent of regular smokers with at least a college degree who were able to stop smoking. A 2005 study in *Nicotine & Tobacco Research* found that both education and income were related to cessation attempts and the ability to remain smoke-free for at least three months.

In a 2006 study in the *American Journal of Health Behavior,* researchers also found that education was related to smoking cessation. Data for this study came from patients at a tobacco-dependence treatment center who wanted to quit smoking. The program offered free counseling and nicotine-replacement medications for patients with lower incomes. Therefore, the ability to pay for services was not an issue. Individuals with only high school diplomas were less likely to remain smoke-free than those who had started or completed college. Individuals with a college degree were more likely to abstain from smoking than those with a high school education (or GED). After four weeks, 58.3 percent of people with college educations had still abstained from smoking. Only 35 percent of those with a high school degree were still smoke-free. After 26 weeks, 39.9 percent of those with college educations were still smoke-free, compared to 23.3 percent of patients with a high school diploma.

Fact Or Fiction?

People in the lower social classes have the same access to cessation products as those in the upper classes.

The Facts: With the development of quitlines, money or access to products is less of an obstacle when it comes to smoking cessation. State and federally funded quitlines are available in all 50 states and offer smokers free over-the-phone counseling, and many quitlines provide smoking-cessation products free of charge, such as nicotine replacement therapies. Counselors provide smokers with support and strategies to stop smoking.

In a 2004 study in the *American Journal of Public Health,* researchers found no socioeconomic differences in quit attempts. However, those within higher socioeconomic groups were more likely to successfully become former smokers. This means that smokers of all socioeconomic groups attempt to quit, but those in the higher groups are more successful.

SOCIOECONOMIC STATUS AND TOBACCO MARKETING

Tobacco companies heavily market products to lower socioeconomic groups. The companies understand the socioeconomic differences in smoking behavior, It makes financial sense to market to the lower socioeconomic classes because they are more likely to start and continue smoking. Tobacco industry documents refer to the lower classes as the "downscale market." An internal document from R.J. Reynolds described the downscale market as: "less educated, are into escapism because they have no intellectual diversions, more malleable, always looking for instant gratification, have nothing to look forward to, and kids see themselves as grownups. These groups live in the moment and do not worry about the long-term consequences of smoking."

In a 2005 study in *Tobacco Control,* the authors show how tobacco companies tailor their marketing messages to different populations. Cigarette companies in India used different imagery when marketing to different social classes. The overall goal was to convey that smoking and success go hand-in-hand. Advertisements to the upper classes used Western images that clearly conveyed success. For the lower classes, more abstract images of smoking and success were used. More concrete images were used for the upper classes because success is a way of life for that group. No imagination is needed to know what it means to be successful. On the other hand, members of the lower classes are often not considered especially successful. They do not know what it means to have an abundance of money, a nice home or automobile, and so forth. Using abstract images allows members of these classes to use their imagination and visualize how success and smoking go together.

Tobacco companies have also marketed cigarettes to the homeless and mentally ill. In a 2005 study in *Tobacco Control,* authors reviewed tobacco industry documents and found companies actively marketed to these groups. The documents showed that companies would donate cigarettes to organizations that served the homeless. Company-branded supplies were also donated to the homeless. The documents indicate that Philip Morris distributed blankets that were labeled with the "Merit" brand to the homeless and shelters. Because social-service organizations are always in need of donations, they welcome the offers made by tobacco companies.

Research has shown that tobacco companies also advertise more in poorer neighborhoods than wealthier ones. In a 2002 study in *Tobacco Control,* researchers examined the number of advertisements around various parts of Boston. Poorer neighborhoods had significantly more storefront tobacco advertisements than wealthier neighborhoods. The authors also discovered that advertisements for menthol cigarettes were heavily marketed in African-American and Latino neighborhoods. This is important because menthol cigarettes are usually the cigarettes of choice by new smokers.

See also: Advertising and Smoking; Cost of Smoking; Quitting, Therapies for

FURTHER READING
Krueger, Hans, Dan Williams, Barbara Kaminsky, and David McLean. *The Health Impact of Smoking and Obesity and What to Do About It.* Toronto, Ontario: University of Toronto Press, 2007.
Lloyd, Barbara. *Smoking in Adolescence: Images and Identities.* New York: Routledge, 1998.

■ TOBACCO WORLDWIDE

Consumers in other countries choose among competing local cigarette brands. In still others, people purchase brands produced by the **transnational** tobacco companies, with operations and sales in many countries. These brand names are familiar to most Americans. They are the same brands that dominate the tobacco market in the United States.

To consider the scale of the worldwide tobacco business, it might be helpful to consider the following: According to the United States Department of Agriculture (USDA), there were 484 billion cigarettes produced in 2006. The USDA also estimates that 5.53 trillion cigarettes were produced worldwide in 2004.

While smoking has declined in the United States, Canada, most of the western and northern European nations, and in Japan, it is still increasing in many eastern European countries, the Russian republics, China, and most countries in the developing world. The American Cancer Society reports that in some developing countries, smoking rates are as high as 50 percent for the male population. Rates for women are generally lower, about 9 percent. However, thanks to advertisements targeting women, the number of female smokers is rising in countries such as Cambodia, Malaysia, and Bangladesh.

In 2000, there were five million deaths worldwide from diseases related to smoking, divided roughly equally between developed and developing nations. That number is certain to rise in the future. Many countries are just beginning to reach the highest U.S. male smoking rate (51.9 percent in 1964). In the 1980s, 20 years after that high point, American cancer deaths rose steeply. If the same situation repeats itself, the world cancer rate will undergo an unprecedented rise in the 2020s.

Even if male smoking rates begin to decline now, there will still be millions, maybe hundreds of millions, of tobacco-related deaths in future decades. Although some observers believe the decline is about to begin, smoking still seems to be on the rise.

Consider China, with the largest smoking population in the world— 350 million out of a population of 1.2 billion. China produces and consumes 30 percent of the world's cigarettes. In the 1980s, Chinese smokers consumed 12 cigarettes a day. By 1996, daily consumption rose to 16 cigarettes per smoker per day, comparable to the 22 daily cigarettes smoked on average by smokers in industrialized countries.

The tobacco habit is heavily tilted toward males in China. Two-thirds of adult males smoke but only 3 percent of females do. Presently, tobacco-related diseases kill one million Chinese a year. If death rates for cancer, cardiovascular disease, and respiratory ailments remain the same, as many as 100 million Chinese men under age 30 may die prematurely.

WHO ARE THE MAJOR COMPETITORS?

Some 100 countries around the world produce tobacco. China leads, growing 5.18 billion pounds per year. The United States comes second, producing 1.323 billion pounds, followed by India (1.156 billion pounds) and Brazil (877 million pounds).

The real powers in the tobacco industry are not the growers but the producers of tobacco products, mainly cigarettes. Operating in a number of countries, these transnational corporations buy tobacco from farmers around the world, manufacture it into various products, and then ship and market their products globally. Several of these major companies are American, such as R.J. Reynolds and Philip Morris, or British, like the British American Tobacco Company. Although the United States ranks second in tobacco production, it's number one when it comes to exporting finished products (that is, cigarettes). The United States ties with Brazil in exporting tobacco leaves to other countries.

Actions by the major cigarette makers to shift production facilities to other countries have led to a steady decline in American cigarette exports since 1997. Manufacturing cigarettes in countries with lower wages has added to the profits of American tobacco companies.

The transnational companies have also engaged in massive programs to encourage farmers in developing countries to grow tobacco.

Almost 75 percent of the land devoted to tobacco growing is found in developing nations. In some, tobacco makes a significant contribution to the national economy. Tobacco leaves account for 6 percent of Malawi's exports and 23 percent of Zimbabwe's. This trade brings much-needed foreign currency into these countries. For many nations, however, the cost of importing American-style cigarettes is much higher than the profits received from exporting tobacco leaves. These countries actually lose on the trade.

Fact Or Fiction?

The tobacco companies and tobacco farmers always pull together when people attack cigarettes.

The Facts: Actually, the tobacco companies have been dealing less with tobacco farmers in recent years. Thanks to tobacco farms they've developed in other countries, cheaper imported tobacco makes up almost one-half of what's inside today's "American" cigarettes. In the American tobacco market, prices have dropped and so has production. This means hard economic times for these farmers.

IMPACT ON GLOBAL ECONOMY

When asked about their operations in various countries, the transnational corporations like to point out the benefits to the host nations. According to a 2003 release on British American Tobacco's South African web site, the tobacco trade benefits 150 countries around the world. The industry supports farmers and workers in many countries, while paying taxes to many national governments. Tobacco is grown on less than 0.3 percent of the world's farmland. Because it grows well in poor soils and under difficult weather conditions, it provides farmers with a stable cash crop. Because of the relatively high profit, farmers can use small tobacco plots to raise money for other farming efforts.

Critics paint a less glowing picture. Because tobacco depletes nutrients in the soil, farmers become dependent on expensive fertilizers to restore their fields. In many cases, foreign currency credits created by tobacco exports are wiped out by the costs of importing the finished product—cigarettes.

As for the tax benefits governments enjoy from the tobacco business, these must be balanced against public health costs from illnesses caused by tobacco smoking. The American Cancer Society estimates that the five million smoking-related deaths of 2003 will balloon to 10 million a year by 2030. The World Health Organization estimates that more than 80 percent of tobacco-related deaths will be in low- and middle-income countries by 2030.

NEW MARKETS

With a high percentage of males already smoking around the world, tobacco companies target ad campaigns at women and (where the local culture allows it) children. This marketing effort has been going on since the 1980s in East Asia and Southeast Asia, in countries like South Korea, Japan, Cambodia, Taiwan, Malaysia, and Bangladesh.

A 2003 report by the American Cancer Society, the World Health Organization (the public health agency of the United Nations), and the International Union Against Cancer (the world's only global anticancer organization), offered a country by country look at tobacco use and tobacco control. In developing countries, tobacco companies have introduced cigarette brands and advertising specifically for women. Cigarette companies sponsor beauty pageants, female sporting events, and even women's social and political organizations to reach their targeted markets. In some Pacific island nations like Nauru, the Cook Islands, and Papua New Guinea, female smokers now outnumber men. This phenomenon has also been noted in developed countries like Sweden. In Denmark, Ireland, and the United Kingdom, 15- and 16-year-old girls are now more likely than boys to become smokers.

When governments have tried to control tobacco imports for economic or health reasons, as in Thailand, American tobacco companies have not hesitated to ask U.S. government agencies for help. The 1974 Trade Act, a law designed to punish countries like Japan for refusing to import American-made cars, was used instead to threaten countries that did not want American cigarettes. Transnational companies also rely on various organizations for fostering trade to open markets and remove bans on cigarette advertising and promotion.

In 2000, the World Health Organization began to consider the problems tobacco can cause around the world. After three years of negotiation, 40 nations signed the world's first global public health treaty, the Framework Convention on Tobacco Control. This agreement sets out regulations for the contents of tobacco products, packaging, labeling, advertising and promotion, smuggling, taxes, and effects on the environment. The intent is to protect developing nations in their dealings with the large tobacco companies. As of 2008, the United States has not ratified this treaty.

Q & A

Question: My friend has been smoking some foreign cigarettes lately. They come in different flavors, and he says he's really enjoying them. What's the story on them?

Answer: These foreign smokes could be clove cigarettes or bidis, hand-rolled cigarettes from India that come in flavors that attract young people, like cherry, chocolate, strawberry, or vanilla. However, these products also have more nicotine and release more carbon monoxide and tar than regular cigarettes. These products may look like fun to smoke, but they are actually more dangerous. You may want to warn your friend before he finds himself with an even harder habit to control.

THE EFFECT ON THE UNITED STATES

The North Carolina Department of Agriculture and Consumer Services reports that there are 662,000 tobacco-related jobs in the United States. In North Carolina alone, there are 255,000 tobacco-related jobs. These jobs are most directly associated with tobacco—growing the plants and manufacturing cigarettes.

In 2002, the average cigarette manufacturing job paid $26.88 an hour. By comparison, the average manufacturing job paid $15.29 an hour. However, through automation and by opening new plants overseas, tobacco companies have been steadily eliminating these high-paying positions. From a high of 46,000 manufacturing jobs in 1983, the number of cigarette workers declined to 26,000 in 1999 and 19,624 by 2006.

International tobacco buying by the cigarette companies has caused prices in the American tobacco market to drop steeply. The downturn has affected the southern states where most tobacco is grown. For the five major tobacco states, the 2005 harvests generated $294 million in Kentucky, $413 million in North Carolina, $62 million in South Carolina, $61 million in Virginia, and $97 million in Tennessee. By comparison, the 2002 harvest in Tennessee brought $155 million.

ISSUES

According to the government's 2002 Census of Agriculture, 37,013 farms grew tobacco. These ranged from large-scale agricultural businesses to family operations with a small field devoted to tobacco on a cattle or crop farm. However, the income from that tobacco may mean the difference between a profit or a loss for a family. For 70 percent of farmers, tobacco brings in about $20,000 a year. The rest of the farmers' income comes from other crops or working at jobs away from the farm.

An acre of tobacco can bring in approximately $4,000. Farmers would need seven acres of cotton or 67 acres of soybeans to match that profit. Those crops need to be irrigated. Nonirrigated peanuts would need 88 acres.

However, the price of tobacco and the size of harvests have been going down as a result of competition from cheap imported tobacco. American cigarette and tobacco interests have invested heavily to promote tobacco farming in numerous developing nations. They then import this cheaper tobacco for use in cigarettes. In 1970, only 16 percent of the tobacco used in American cigarettes came from abroad. In 2005, the proportion was 55.9 percent.

As part of the Master Settlement Agreement (MSA) resulting from lawsuits filed by the states against the major tobacco corporations, the companies agreed to set up a fund to help tobacco farmers. Over 12 years, $5.15 billion will be distributed to tobacco-growing states.

REPLACEMENT PRODUCTS

In addition to the money directly earmarked for farmers in the tobacco settlement, a number of states are using other payments from the MSA to develop alternatives to the tobacco business. North Carolina's Golden LEAF Foundation invested part of the state's tobacco settlement in a new industrial site. In most states, however, the concentration is on improving roads and services in poorer, tobacco-dependent counties and on finding alternative crops.

Virginia State University and Virginia Tech have evaluated more than 30 various crops that can replace tobacco. Tobacco farmers in Kentucky are experimenting with chickens that run free instead of being cooped and dairy farming, including cheese-making. North

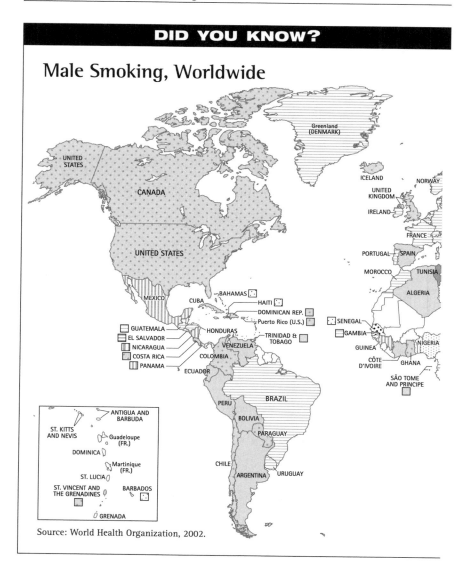

DID YOU KNOW?

Male Smoking, Worldwide

Source: World Health Organization, 2002.

Carolina farmers are switching to vegetables like lettuce, broccoli, and Chinese cabbage.

Some farmers have established partnerships with Community Supported Agriculture. This program allows families in cities to invest in farms, paying for operations and salary and getting part of the crop—fresh, safe produce—in return.

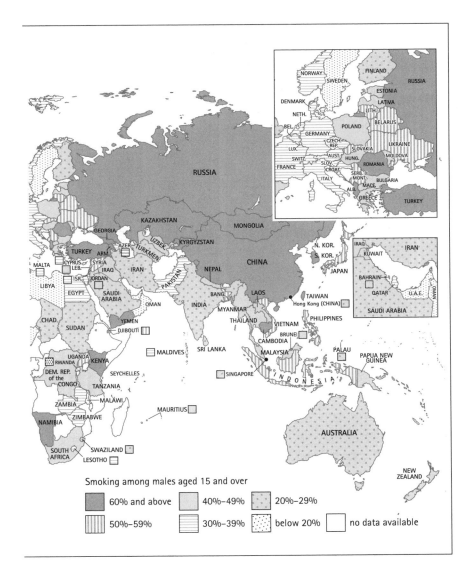

Smoking among males aged 15 and over

- 60% and above
- 50%–59%
- 40%–49%
- 30%–39%
- 20%–29%
- below 20%
- no data available

While younger farmers may gamble on developing alternative crops, older farmers may find it too difficult to switch. These farmers may also find it too expensive to continue growing tobacco. Between 1954 and 1992, the number of tobacco farms dropped by 75 percent. From 1992 to 1998, an additional 35,000 small tobacco farms disappeared. According to the United States Department of

Agriculture, 56,977 farms grew tobacco in 2002. This is down from 93,530 tobacco-growing farms in 1997. This is a 39 percent decrease in five years.

GLOBAL BUSINESS, LOCAL PROBLEMS

For more than two decades, the major cigarette manufacturers have-been expanding their operations to nations around the world. The companies buy tobacco in 100 countries, many of them developing nations where the transnational corporations have encouraged production. Manufacturing plants have also been set up overseas, in countries where labor is cheaper and health regulations less troublesome.

As globalization continues in the tobacco industry, American workers and farmers in the tobacco business will continue to suffer declines.

See also: Government and Tobacco; Smoking and Society; Smoking, History of

FURTHER READING

Gately, Iain. *Tobacco.* New York: Grove Press, 2002.

Parker, Philip M. *The World Market for Stripped and Stemmed Tobacco: A 2007 Global Trade Perspective.* San Diego, Calif.: ICON Group International, 2006.

■ WEIGHT, SELF-IMAGE, AND SMOKING

See: Media and Smoking, The; Women and Smoking

■ WITHDRAWAL

A condition that results from the abrupt ending of a dependency-inducing drug, such as tobacco, is called withdrawal. Symptoms include anxiety, a bad temper, restlessness and difficulty concentrating, depression, tingling in the hands and feet, sweating, intestinal disorders, headaches, coughing, sore throats, coldlike symptoms, and strong desires for cigarettes.

According to the CDC, 31.7 million of the nation's 45.3 million smokers in 2006 wanted to quit. Yet few people who try to stop smoking are successful in their attempt. The Centers for Disease Control and Prevention (CDC) estimates that only 5 percent succeed by going "cold turkey"—just stopping on their own. While pro-smoking advocates talk about willpower and people being too eager to call themselves victims, the question of **nicotine** addiction also must be considered.

SYMPTOMS

Whenever a person with an addiction stops taking the habit-forming substance, he or she experiences withdrawal symptoms. The human body learns to live with a certain dosage of heroin, cocaine, or nicotine. This process is called **tolerance**. In fact, often the body needs more and more of the substance to feel normal. When the substance is removed, the body will suffer until it gets used to operating without a drug. With heroin, withdrawal symptoms can be so painful and dangerous that they become life-threatening.

Nicotine withdrawal is not as dangerous. But the symptoms, taken together, can make people so miserable that they'll light up again as the easy way out.

Nicotine stimulates the brain's pleasure centers. It creates other effects that can be considered positive by the user. Nicotine helps people concentrate, especially in noisy surroundings. It helps users to deal with stress and can also prevent feelings of depression.

One set of withdrawal symptoms might be considered the reverse of nicotine's "positive" effects. Instead of managing stress with cigarettes, people can become more anxious and irritable when they try to quit. They may also have a harder time concentrating and thinking. People trying to quit the nicotine habit also complain of feeling sad or depressed. Some compare their attempts to quit smoking as similar to losing a good friend.

Those striving to give up smoking often find themselves feeling hungry. Nicotine depresses the appetite. So people who quit often gain weight—about five pounds on average, though women have been known to gain more.

As some smokers try to quit, they also experience a sudden loss of energy. Nicotine stimulates production of the hormone epinephrine, a chemical that revs up the body. Fatigue can set in once the body is deprived of its nicotine dose.

Another set of withdrawal symptoms can be attributed to the physical effects of tar, nicotine, and the other irritating chemicals in cigarette smoke. Some people complain of coughs, runny noses, and even sore throats when they quit the habit. While they smoked, their bodies had to create extra mucus to carry away smoke particles. It takes a little time for that extra production to wind down. The final surge of mucus may be compared to spring cleaning in the body. The moist membranes in the nose and throat are getting rid of irritants that built up during the time the person was smoking. The lungs are also cleaning themselves, expelling all the tar that was deposited on the tissues.

Other physical symptoms of withdrawal include headaches, dizziness, and tingling in the hands and feet. These symptoms show that the cardiovascular system is recovering from the effects of nicotine. When people start smoking, chemicals in the smoke cause the blood vessels to constrict, cutting off the blood supply. They also breathe in poisonous carbon monoxide, which interferes with the oxygen supply in the blood. The result is that new smokers often feel dizzy.

When a person stops smoking, the situation reverses itself. Blood vessels relax, allowing increased blood flow. The blood itself is more oxygenated. The body can respond to this as a "rush," so that the former smoker feels light-headed and dizzy.

Worst of all from the former smoker's point of view are the sudden and powerful attacks of **craving** for a cigarette. Such flare-ups can grow in intensity until they're almost unbearable. Sometimes cravings can be associated with activities or feelings that led a person to smoke. For instance, a person who used to have a cigarette after dinner may be hit by a craving at that time. A person who felt awkward in social settings might have lit a cigarette to give his hands something to do. A person going through a stressful experience might use a cigarette as a way to calm down.

At other times, cravings seem to come from nowhere or may be triggered by almost subliminal cues. Former smokers recall cravings after smelling cigarette smoke, seeing a lit cigarette in an ashtray, or even feeling a cigarette in their hands.

Part of these sudden desires is physical, the need for nicotine. Part of the problem is psychological, the struggle to break a habit. People become used to having a cigarette in their mouths. They grow accustomed to having a cigarette in their hands and going through the rituals of smoking. Without these habits, many find themselves on edge, so that the smallest trigger can result in a huge attack on their willpower.

Fact Or Fiction?

These health statistics they announce are just a lot of meaningless numbers to scare people into quitting.

The Facts: When it comes to a serious national problem, the numbers are going to be large. The idea that 438,000 people will die from tobacco-related illnesses and conditions every year is mind-boggling. But consider the families slowly losing a grandfather or grandmother to agonizing cancer. Think of the young people facing the untimely death of an uncle, an aunt . . . or parent. In terms of the human costs, these statistics have a very personal—and painful—meaning.

WEAPONS AGAINST CRAVING

Some people attempting to quit the habit just grit their teeth and suffer through cravings. Others, in spite of good intentions, give in and go back to smoking.

Psychological techniques can be helpful to avoid cravings or deal with them. A quit diary, begun well before the actual quitting date, can be an invaluable tool. Jotting down where and why they smoke and their mental state when they have a cigarette can help smokers learn what makes them light up. If possible, they can steer clear of many of these triggers. If not, they will at least be prepared. Another psychological technique is the practice of timing the length of a craving. Cravings can build in intensity until they seem unstoppable, but like a wave, they pass. Being aware of how long they have to withstand a craving helps strengthen the will to resist them.

Another way to deal with cravings is through nicotine replacement therapy. A variety of products are now available, both over-the-counter and with a doctor's prescription. The nicotine patch transmits a constant low dose of nicotine through the skin to help blunt cravings while people attempt to quit. Nicotine gum, lozenges, and nasal sprays are also used to maintain a basic dose, but these treatments offer the chance of taking an additional dose to defeat a craving.

The strategy behind nicotine replacement is to lower the dose of nicotine until the person is entirely free. The recommended length of the treatment is eight to 12 weeks, though some people have remained on replacement therapy for six months. Combined with psychological and behavioral help, nicotine replacement therapy can attain a success rate between 25 to 33 percent of users remaining smoke-free six months after their quit date. That compares with a success rate of 5 to 6 percent for people using willpower alone.

Drug therapy is also available for those who wish to quit smoking. Buproprion, a medication originally developed to help against depression, has proven effective in dealing with withdrawal symptoms, especially cravings. Marketed under the name Zyban, it is available with a doctor's prescription.

Smokers considering any of these therapies, including over-the-counter ones, should consult a doctor first. They should discuss any medical conditions and present medications to make sure the new therapies will not create any risks to their health.

Q & A

Question: Ever since I stopped smoking, I find myself fidgeting all the time. I was never the nervous type before. Is there something wrong with me?

Answer: Unfortunately, you're going through another normal nicotine withdrawal symptom. Look on the bright side: you're not feeling dizzy or knocked out.

The best thing you can do is to find some way to distract your body. Exercise may help. Besides giving you something to do, it will help clean out your system.

CHEATING AND REPEATING

Smoking while trying to quit not only defeats the purpose of nicotine replacement or medication but can also be dangerous. A 1996 study by Duke University found that those who cheated on the first day of quitting were overwhelmingly more likely to remain smokers six months later. If the success rate using the nicotine patch was approximately one in four, the success rate for the cheaters was one in 40.

Smokers who try but fail to quit should not dismiss the effort. Rather, they should chalk it up to experience and see what they can learn from the attempt. *The Health Benefits of Smoking Cessation*, a 1990 report by the **surgeon general**, the nation's leading public health official, noted that success in quitting smoking requires a number of attempts.

In a 2008 study in *Nicotine and Tobacco Research*, investigators found that smokers who made an attempt to quit and failed were more likely to reduce tobacco consumption. They also found that 52 percent reduced their consumption, although 22 percent increased it.

The good news for anyone trying to beat the habit is that the worst withdrawal symptoms ease within 48 to 72 hours after that last cigarette. The National Institute on Drug Abuse (NIDA) says that most withdrawal symptoms will diminish within a few weeks. However, the NIDA web site warns that for some people, it can take months or longer before they are completely symptom-free.

See also: Addiction to Nicotine; Body and Smoking, The; Addiction, Products to Overcome; Quitting, Therapies for

FURTHER READING
Brizer, David. *Quitting Smoking for Dummies.* New York: Wiley, 2003.
Whetherall, Charles. *Quit: Read This Book and Stop Smoking.* Philadelphia: Running Press Miniature Editions, 2007.

■ WOMEN AND SMOKING

While women had been growing tobacco and even manufacturing tobacco products since colonial times, few women smoked it until the 1920s. For generations, British and later American society frowned on the idea of female tobacco use. This strong disapproval held until well into the 1800s. In the early 1900s, tobacco companies began looking for new markets for their product. Lucky Strike and other brands aimed their advertising at women. Rates of female smoking rose not only in the 1920s but also in the 1930s, 1940s, and 1950s. At the height of the smoking boom in the mid-1960s, almost one-third of women smoked.

TEENS SPEAK

I Fell for the Image

Gabrielle is 17, a high school junior. She started smoking when she was 15.

"When I was younger, I thought about becoming a model. Whenever I saw a fashion magazine, I just tore right through it.

"You might say that cigarettes started out as an accessory for me. I'd see these tall, graceful women, and in their hands there'd be a cigarette. So I began trying them. I wouldn't say they made me taller or more graceful. But I did think they made me look older and maybe cooler.

"That was the way things looked in the mirror. Outside, though, smoking could be a hassle. I could smoke at some friends' houses, but not at others. Our local mall doesn't allow smoking at all.

"As for school, well, don't even think about smoking. We can't even do it on the school grounds. If you want to smoke, you have to do it across the way, behind a supermarket. I'll just say this—it's not too elegant. There are all these smells from rotting food. We might as well be smoking in a dumpster.

"I was standing outside, freezing, with the other kids who smoked the other day. A bunch of kids from school passed by, and they were laughing at us!"

THE NUMBERS

Fewer women smoke today than men. After news about the health risks of smoking became well-known, smoking declined for both sexes. In 1965, 51.9 percent of men smoked. That figure fell to 25.2 percent in 2001, more than a 50 percent drop. Among women, however, the percentage of smokers went from 33.9 to 20.7 percent, a reduction of less than 40 percent. Fewer women quit smoking than men. In 2006, 23.9 percent of men smoked, while 18 percent of women smoked.

The American Lung Association reports that in 2003, 48.8 percent of women tried to quit smoking for at least one day.

A 2001 study for the National Institute on Drug Abuse (NIDA) suggests that women may associate more situations and moods with smoking, creating more triggers for cigarette cravings. The study also found that the nicotine replacement therapy was less effective because women's body chemistry shifts more than men's due to menstruation, the monthly process among women of childbearing age in which the lining of the uterus is shed. The process is controlled by the interaction of a number of body chemicals called hormones.

The National Cancer Institute (NCI) estimates that there will be 215,020 new cases of lung cancer in 2008. Males will account for 114,690 of these new cases, while females will account for the remaining 100,330 cases. The NCI also predicts that 161,840 people will die from lung cancer in 2008. Women will account for 71,030 of these deaths. In January of 2004, researchers at the Weill Cornell Medical Center in New York studied computed tomography (CT) scans of patients for structural abnormalities. These computer-enhanced X-ray images showed that female smokers were 2.7 times more likely to develop lung cancer than men who smoked the same amount. In April 2004, researchers at Northwestern University in Chicago announced that lung cancer is an entirely different disease in men and women, because of differences in women's body structure and growth, physical processes, and body chemistry. They also pointed out that the rate of lung cancer in women had increased 600 percent between 1930 and 1997, rising 60 percent between 1990 and 2003. The rise was termed "an epidemic."

These discoveries supplement earlier work by the CDC that examined data from 1995 to 1999 on life expectancy for smokers. Male smokers lived 13.2 years less than nonsmokers. Females lived 14.5 years less than their nonsmoking counterparts.

A possible reason for a woman's greater risk of developing lung cancer may be genetic. Genes make up the instruction book for the body, regulating the growth of bodily structures and their functions. Animal studies in 2004 found that female mice lacked a functioning gene involved in the creation of a particular enzyme, a body chemical that triggers chemical reactions. The enzyme creates a reaction that kills cancerous cells. Questions still remain over whether women may lack a gene that helps clean out carcinogens or repairs genetic damage from cancer-causing chemicals in cigarette smoke.

Fact Or Fiction?

When it comes to cancer, breast cancer is the one women have to worry about.

The Facts: In 1987, lung cancer became the number one killer of American women. The disease has held this slot for more than 21 years. Yet 80 percent of women still mistakenly believe that breast cancer is their most serious cancer risk.

THE TEENAGE ISSUE

Tobacco companies are often criticized for advertisements to capture young smokers. With the declining numbers of adult smokers, recruitment of "replacement smokers" among young people remains an important business strategy.

Teen smoking spiked upward in the 1990s but declined again by 2001. In the 2007 Youth Risk Behavior Survey, researchers report that 48.8 percent of girls had ever tried a cigarette. Only 11.8 percent of girls either currently smoked daily or had smoked daily at some point in their lives.

Why do teenage girls start smoking? They're in a time of life when questions of image are very important. An important part of a girl's image is influenced by body types shown in the media. Slim, athletic, attractive figures are the ideal, but hard to match in reality. In a 2006 study in *Nutrition Journal,* the authors found that smoking is one strategy female college students use to lose weight. In this study, 9 percent of females admitted to this practice. In a 2006 study in *Addictive Behavior*, authors found that women believed smoking was an effective weight-loss strategy. While smoking does have an effect on appetite, it's a small benefit to weigh against so many future dangers.

Q & A

Question: My friend has been talking about quitting smoking for a while. Now she's getting serious, and she's asked for my help. What can I do?

Answer: Your friend is smart to look for support. Quitting can be hard for teenagers, especially girls. Talk to your friend and find out what you can do to help.

Maybe you'll want to check in with her more often, not to see how the quitting attempt is going, but just to be a friend. She may have more need for a friendly ear.

Be encouraging. You may want to think of small rewards for celebrating a week or a month without smoking. It might be as simple as a free movie or dinner at a nonsmoking restaurant. Be creative, be fun, but most of all, be there for your friend.

INTERACTION WITH BIRTH CONTROL

Oral contraception, or the pill, is the most popular form of birth control in the United States. Birth control pills prevent the creation of a baby by stopping a woman's ovaries from releasing an egg. The pill does this by combining two hormones found in the body to work on the ovary. Oral contraception is 92 to 99 percent effective, with few problems for healthy women.

However, risks have been discovered for women age 35 and over who smoke. Blood clots may form, which can block blood vessels and cause heart attacks and strokes. In a 2003 study released in the British medical magazine *The Lancet,* researchers examined the health records of 17,000 women and found that older patients who smoked and used birth control pills were two to three times as likely to die from heart disease. A 2001 study in the *New England Journal of Medicine* found that the lower-dose birth control pills used in recent years lower the risk of heart attack—except for women who smoke, have high cholesterol, or high blood pressure.

The best advice for women using oral contraceptives? Don't smoke.

PREGNANCY

When a pregnant woman smokes, she exposes the fetus, the unborn infant, to a number of cancer-causing chemicals and poisons. As a fact sheet from the Centers for Disease Control and Prevention (CDC) warns, pregnant smokers face a risk of miscarrying or going into premature labor.

Children born to smoking mothers have a lower birth weight. However, if the mother stops smoking when she discovers she's pregnant or three to four months into the pregnancy, the risk of having a low-birth-weight baby falls to the same percentages as nonsmoking mothers.

The CDC also warns that women who smoke while pregnant are at greater risk of losing the baby before his or her first birthday. Infants born to mothers who smoked in pregnancy are more likely to die of SIDS (sudden infant death syndrome), a medical condition in which seemingly healthy babies die in their sleep.

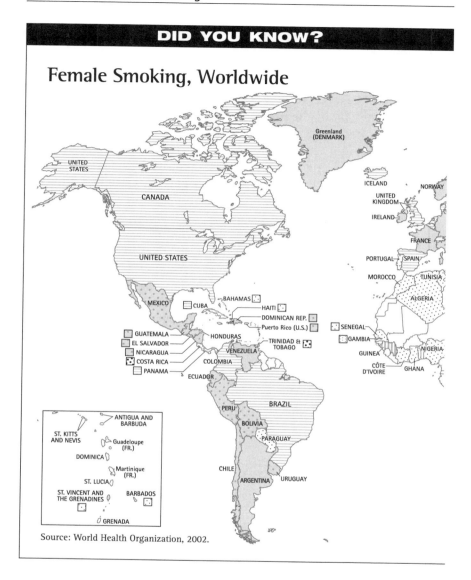

DID YOU KNOW?

Female Smoking, Worldwide

Source: World Health Organization, 2002.

As the children of women who smoked during pregnancy grow older, they may fall behind in physical growth and intellectual development. Dr. Peter Fried, a Canadian researcher who has followed children whose mothers smoked in pregnancy since 1980, identified three measurable problems in a 1999 report. The children were slower in developing speech, they suffered from impulsive

Smoking among females aged 15 and over

- ||| 40%–49%
- ▨ 30%–39%
- ▤ 20%–29%
- ⋰ 10%–19%
- ⋰ below 10%
- ☐ no data available

behavior or hyperactivity, and they scored slightly lower in intelligence testing.

Expectant mothers are beginning to understand some of these dangers. In 2005, 12.4 percent of pregnant women age 15 to 44 smoked. About 40 percent of all women in that age group smoked. Only 25 percent of smoking women stopped during pregnancy to protect their children.

MENOPAUSE

Menopause marks the end of a woman's child-bearing years. Many changes take place in the body and with the body's chemistry. Considering the large number of chemicals in cigarette smoke, it should be no surprise that smoking might affect this phase of a woman's life.

A 2001 study at Massachusetts General Hospital in Boston entitled "Smoking Likely to Trigger Earlier Menopause" affirmed what many doctors had noted about female patients who smoked. The Boston researchers identified a chemical in cigarette smoke that kills eggs in the ovaries. Women are born with only a limited lifetime supply of eggs and face the onset of menopause as this supply runs low. The damage caused by cigarette smoke can go unnoticed for years, until a woman suddenly has no fertile eggs left. Such unexpected, premature menopause can be a problem for women who decided to wait to have children until after establishing a career.

Osteoporosis is a condition that concerns many older women. As women age, their bones become thinner, often breaking. A broken leg or hip can leave otherwise healthy women housebound. Studies have shown that smoking seems to accelerate the bone loss.

Studies from the 1980s showed that smoking works on the body to reduce estrogen, a female hormone. This reduction may play a part in the onset of early menopause as well as osteoporosis. Medical experts advise those diagnosed with osteoporosis to stop smoking. Treatment for the condition includes calcium supplements, weight-bearing exercise, drugs, and hormone replacement therapy.

The health risks of smoking would seem to be enough to deter any woman from smoking. Yet large numbers of young women take up the habit every year, a striking example of the success of advertising.

DAUGHTERS OF WOMEN WHO SMOKE

Children whose parents smoke have a greater chance of becoming smokers themselves. According to some sources, these young people are twice as likely to pick up the habit.

In a 1998 study in the *Journal of Research on Adolescence*, researchers found that mothers who smoked during pregnancy were more likely to have daughters who smoked. If a mother smoked during pregnancy, daughters were 3.8 times more likely to smoke daily within the past year. The researchers raised the possibility that nicotine in the expecting mother's bloodstream somehow "primed" the brain of the unborn baby to react to the drug later in life. Sons did not show the same willingness to pick up the smoking habit. The authors of the study theorized that male body chemicals called hormones somehow interfered with the effect of nicotine on unborn boys.

However, a 1997 study by researchers from the University of Chicago and the University of Pittsburgh did find an effect of smoking during pregnancy on boys. The researchers were studying the backgrounds of boys being counseled for conduct disorder, a pattern of continued antisocial behavior that includes lying, fighting, vandalism, and fire-setting. Of the mothers who had smoked a half a pack per day during pregnancy, 80 percent had sons with conduct problems. For nonsmoking mothers, the rate was 50 percent.

Another Columbia study in 1999 showed that sons whose mothers smoked in pregnancy showed greater conduct problems, while daughters were five times more likely to fall into a substance abuse problem during their teen years.

A six-year study from the University of Chicago on disruptive boys found that sons whose mothers smoked half a pack of cigarettes per day during pregnancy were exhibiting conduct problems five times beyond the general population by the time the boys were seven years old.

While the mechanism that sets up these behavior problems, both for males and females, has yet to be identified, the studies definitely establish that there is a problem and that it represents another long-term effect of smoking during pregnancy.

See also: Advertising and Smoking; Media and Smoking, The

FURTHER READING

Gately, Iain. *Tobacco.* New York: Grove Press, 2002.
Tolson, Katherine P., and Emily B. Veksler. *Research Focus on Smoking and Women's Health.* Hauppauge, N.Y.: Nova Science Publishers, 2008.

HOTLINES AND HELP SITES

Action on Smoking and Health (ASH)
URL: http://www.ash.org
Phone: 1-202-659-4310
Mission: A national nonprofit legal action and educational organization fighting for the rights of nonsmokers against the many problems of smoking
Programs: Offers news summaries and fact sheets on a number of subjects, including teen smoking, secondhand smoke, and nicotine addiction

American Cancer Society
URL: http://www.cancer.org
Phone: 1-800-ACS-2345 (1-800-227-2345)
National Quitline: 1-877-YES-QUIT (1-877-937-7848)
Mission: A nationwide community-based voluntary health organization dedicated to eliminating cancer as a major health problem
Programs: Provides resources devoted to educating the public about the dangers of tobacco and to advocating laws and regulations regarding sales and advertising of tobacco, especially to young people. The American Cancer Society's national and local quitlines help a large number of smokers who wish to escape the habit.

American Heart Association
URL: http://www.americanheart.org
Phone: 1-800-AHA-USA1 (1-800-242-8721)

Mission: A national voluntary health agency whose mission is to reduce disability and death from cardiovascular diseases and stroke

Programs: Offers public health education about lifestyle choices such as exercise and tobacco control, including numerous articles and fact sheets on the dangers of smoking, as well as useful tips on quitting

American Legacy Foundation

URLs: http://www.americanlegacy.org
http://www.join-the-circle.org
http://www.streetheory.org
http://www.thetruth.com

Phone: 1-202-454-5555

Quitline: 1-800-339-5589

Mission: Dedicated to building a world where young people reject tobacco and anyone can quit

Programs: The foundation was established and funded as a result of the Master Settlement Agreement between state attorneys general and tobacco corporations. Its countermarketing efforts have resulted in the striking truth national advertising campaign, which has stimulated grassroots youth activism. The foundation's Circle of Friends: Uniting to Be Smoke-Free program is a national grassroots social movement to show support for women struggling to quit smoking and to highlight the toll of tobacco-related disease on American women, their families, and communities. The foundation operates a free quitline that offers advice and counseling to Washington, D.C. residents and has a wide range of information available through the above web sites.

American Lung Association (ALA)

URL: http://www.lungusa.org

Phone: 1-800-LUNG-USA (1-800-586-4872)

Mission: The oldest voluntary health organization in the United States, the ALA is today fighting lung disease in all its forms, with special emphasis on asthma, tobacco control, and environmental health

Programs: The ALA has developed Teens Against Tobacco Use (TATU), a peer-teaching tobacco control program aimed at deterring students from taking up smoking. The association also has a smoking cessation program for teens that is called Not On Tobacco, or N-O-T.

Americans for Non-Smokers Rights (ANR)
URL: http://www.no-smoke.org
Phone: 1-510-841-3032
Mission: To create comprehensive programs for youth of all ages on issues of smoking prevention, the benefits of smoke-free air, and the right to breath smoke-free air.
Programs: Provides educational resources for schools, health departments, medical organizations, and others interested in the issues surrounding smoking and secondhand smoke. The ANR also provides educational materials and training seminars for youth and adults to aid in the quest for a smoke-free environment.

Campaign for Tobacco-Free Kids
(National Center for Tobacco-Free Kids)
URL: http://www.tobaccofreekids.org
Phone: 1-202-296-5469 or 1-800-284-KIDS
Mission: to protect children from tobacco addiction and exposure to secondhand smoke
Programs: Campaign for Tobacco-Free Kids is one of the nation's largest nongovernmental initiatives ever launched, working with 130-plus partners (including health, education, medical, civic, corporate, youth, and religious organizations). The center works on national, state, and global tobacco control initiatives, sponsors youth action, issues press releases on tobacco news, and offers research and facts as well as special reports such as Smokeless Tobacco: Don't Be Fooled; Tobacco-Free Schools; and Big Tobacco: Still Addicting Kids

Centers for Disease Control and Prevention's Office on Smoking and Health (OSH)
URL: http://www.cdc.gov/tobacco
Phone: 1-800-CDC-1311
Affiliation: An agency of the Department of Health and Human Services
Mission: To develop and apply disease prevention and control, environmental health, and health promotion

Programs: OSH is responsible for leading and coordinating strategic efforts aimed at preventing tobacco use among youths, promoting smoking cessation among youths and adults, and protecting nonsmokers from environmental tobacco smoke. A variety of publications on smoking, tobacco, and health are available through its toll-free telephone number 24 hours a day; voice recordings of current smoking information and other programs are also available by telephone. The OSH Database, which covers more than 30 years of information and contains more than 60,000 abstracts of scientific and technical literature related to smoking and tobacco use, is used by researchers, librarians, medical professionals, and students nationwide.

New Jersey GASP (Group Against Smoking Pollution)
URL: http://www.njgasp.org
Phone: 1-908-273-9368
Mission: To secure smoke-free air for nonsmokers and ensure tobacco-free lives for children
Programs: Provides information through their web site for out-of-staters on environmental tobacco smoke, suggestions for activists, and a library section with interesting documents, including some pointed comments on banning cigarettes for young people

New Jersey REBEL (Reaching Everyone By Exposing Lies)
URL: http://www.njrebel.com
Phone: 1-732-254-3344
Affiliation: National Council on Alcoholism and Drug Dependence (NCADD)
Mission: To educate and empower youths to make healthy lifestyle decisions and to promote the health and well-being of individuals and communities through the reduction or elimination of alcohol, tobacco, and other substances that cause health problems
Programs: This statewide youth-led antitobacco movement, geared toward students in middle school through high school and going into college, offers facts on tobacco and smoking on both the national and New Jersey levels, with a selection of eye-opening comments from tobacco company memos and documents over the years.

Nicotine Anonymous World Service

URL: http://www.nicotine-anonymous.org

Phone: 1-415-750-0328

Mission: To help all those who would like to cease using tobacco and nicotine products in any form

Programs: Helps people who are seeking freedom from nicotine addiction, including those using cessation programs and nicotine withdrawal aids. The fellowship offers group support and recovery using the 12 Steps as adapted from Alcoholics Anonymous to achieve abstinence from nicotine.

Philip Morris USA

URL: http://www.phillipmorrisusa.com

Affiliation: Philip Morris USA is the American tobacco subsidiary of Altria Group, Inc.

Mission: To communicate openly about the health effects of its products while responsibly marketing them to adults who smoke

Programs: Provides some unexpected data on health issues regarding its products and offers links for more information and help in quitting smoking data

QuitNet

URL: http://www.quitnet.com

Affiliation: Boston University School of Public Health and partnered with the American Legacy Foundation

Mission: To offer a variety of aids to help smokers successfully quit

Programs: Helps smokers map out a personalized quit plan and offers expert advice whenever needed, plus information resources. The web site provides links to an entire community of smokers and ex-smokers to help people quit the habit.

GLOSSARY

acetaldehyde   a chemical created by the burning of sugar; used as an additive in cigarettes

acute disease   an illness that appears suddenly with severe effects

alveoli   small clusters of air sacs in the lungs. Oxygen passes through the thin walls of the alveoli and into the blood, while carbon dioxide passes out of the blood to be exhaled.

ammonia   a chemical used in cigarettes to increase the pH level

atherosclerosis   (also known as hardening of the arteries) a medical condition in which artery walls become less elastic. A thickening in the inside lining of the artery attracts a buildup of material, narrowing the interior of the blood vessel, possibly causing a heart attack or stroke

bidis   flavored cigarettes hand-rolled in India

"Big Tobacco"   the major tobacco corporations in the United States, including Philip Morris, Inc., the R.J. Reynolds Tobacco Company, the Brown & Williamson Tobacco Corporation, the Lorillard Tobacco Company, and the Liggett Group

bronchial tubes   the air passages that connect the trachea (windpipe) and the lungs

calculus (also known as tartar) the difficult-to-remove buildup on the lower parts of the teeth near the gumline

cancer a serious disease in which cells in the body multiply uncontrollably, creating growths which can injure various organs

capillaries very small blood vessels that connect the arteries and veins

carbon monoxide an odorless, colorless poison gas produced by combustion. The gas is present in wood smoke, engine exhaust, and cigarette smoke.

carcinogen a substance that causes cancer

cardiovascular system the heart and the blood vessels, which deliver blood throughout the body. This system brings nutrients and oxygen to all cells while carrying away wastes and carbon dioxide.

catalyst a substance that starts or speeds up a chemical reaction

chemotherapy a medical treatment in which patients receive toxic chemicals to destroy cancer cells

chronic disease an illness that develops or persists over a long period of time

chronic obstructive pulmonary disease (COPD) a lung disease damaging to the lungs, making it hard to breathe

Cigarette Papers, The secret corporate documents from the major tobacco companies, filled with damaging revelations about what the corporations knew about the health and addiction risks of cigarettes

cilia very small hairlike structures growing from the lining of the bronchial tubes, which work to remove debris and foreign bodies from the airway

cold turkey attempting to quit a habit, such as smoking, without tapering off or using other aids

contingency management a strategy for behavioral change consisting of offering rewards for success and punishments for failure

craving an intense desire for an addictive substance

cytokine a body chemical that arouses or suppresses the activity of the body's immune system

dopamine a neurotransmitter released by nerve cells in the limbic region of the brain. This area is associated with feelings of pleasure.

emphysema a medical condition in which the alveoli become enlarged and their walls are destroyed

enzyme a complicated protein created by cells within the body as a catalyst for certain biochemical reactions

"fight or flight" response a physical response that prepares the human body for extreme activity

freebase nicotine a volatile form of nicotine that is rapidly absorbed by the lungs

fuomo loco a genetically altered variety of tobacco containing extremely high amounts of nicotine

genetic having a connection with inherited traits

gingivitis an inflammation of the gums that surround the teeth

halitosis bad breath. Because of the effects of cigarette smoke in the mouth, smokers suffer a particularly strong form of halitosis.

hemoglobin a substance in red blood cells that bonds with oxygen, carrying it to cells where it is needed. The carbon monoxide in cigarette smoke bonds more strongly with hemoglobin than oxygen can, thus reducing the amount of oxygen in the bloodstream.

hormone a body chemical that travels through the bloodstream to change the function of a particular organ

hypnosis an altered state of consciousness where subjects are open to suggestion

hypoxia a shortage of oxygen in the blood

ischemic heart disease a disease characterized by a reduced blood supply to the heart

levulinic acid acid used to reduce the pH level of cigarette smoke

leukoplakia a common, sometimes precancerous, disease of the mouth

lobbying attempting to convince public officials to support your views concerning legislation

lobbyist a representative of a company, industry, or group who attempts to influence lawmakers

Master Settlement Agreement an agreement signed in 1998 to resolve court actions brought by state attorneys general to recover smoking-related costs

Medicaid and **Medicare** nationwide health-care programs specially aimed to help the elderly and the poor. Costs are shared by the federal and state governments.

membrane a thin layer of tissue that surrounds, connects, or separates organs or parts of the body. Mucous membranes line all the passages of the human body that touch air.

menthol a naturally occurring compound that has local anesthetic properties

metastasis the process by which cancer spreads in the body. Cancerous cells break away from tumors and travel through the bloodstream or the lymph system, forming new growths in distant parts of the body.

neurotransmitter a chemical that carries an electrical impulse from a nerve-ending to another nerve or muscle cell

nicotine fading   a smoking cessation method in which the smoker progressively reduces intake of nicotine by smoking brands lower in nicotine

periodontitis   a severe form of **gingivitis** that destroys the soft tissue and bone that support teeth

placebo   a pill containing no medication administered for its psychological effect in medical studies

plaque   a thickened area in the interior wall of an artery. These areas can constrict the flow of blood.

plasma   the clear, yellowish liquid portion of blood

radiation therapy   a medical treatment in which beams of X-rays, electrons, or gamma rays are used to destroy cancer cells within the patient's body, or when radioactive materials are placed in or around a tumor

receptor   a site on the surface of a cell that allows a chemical, such as a neurotransmitter or hormone, to bind to it because the chemical's structure perfectly matches the site

reduced smoking   a method of smoking cessation whereby the smoker gradually reduces the number of cigarettes smoked, first to 50 percent of the original amount, and then stops completely

rehabilitation   medical therapy to restore function to a damaged part of the body

relapse prevention   a behavioral strategy for maintaining a patient's will to change in spite of lapses in changing behavior

remission   a lessening of intensity in a disease. In cancer, an absence of symptoms and evidence of cancer cells in the body

scheduled smoking   a smoking cessation method in which the smoker disrupts habitual smoking patterns by following an arbitrary schedule, gradually extending time periods between cigarettes

securitization   a form of financing involving raising money by offering investors a share of a specific cash flow over time

sedative   a drug that has a tranquilizing effect

smoking cessation   the act of quitting smoking

snuff   a finely powered tobacco that is either inhaled through the nose or used orally

spit tobacco   another, less glamorous, name for smokeless tobacco, often used by antitobacco activists

stimulant   a drug that arouses the activity of the body

stroke   a serious medical condition, usually caused by a blood clot blocking the flow of blood to the brain

subsidy   an amount of money, usually government funds, put up to help an industry or support prices

tar   a residue in cigarette smoke. The solid particles can stick to the tissues of the lungs, causing irritation and serious health problems.

theobromine   a chemical found in cocoa; can be used to dilate blood vessels

tolerance   the process by which the body becomes accustomed to an addictive substance. The body will not respond to a previously effective dose, requiring more of the substance for the addict to feel normal

transnational corporation   (also called multinational) a company with operations in two or more countries

tumor   an abnormal growth that can be cancerous or noncancerous. A cancerous tumor is formed when cells begin dividing wildly.

INDEX

Page numbers in **bold** denote main entries.